Affirmations

1. We accept each other without judgment and are willing to offer and receive mutual caring and support in total confidentiality.

2. We are receptive to new skills and insights.

3. We are open to learning new ways of relating to the elderly.

4. We expect change as part of life; people can learn to understand and handle change.

5. We realize that we cannot control all the circumstances of our lives, nor of our loved ones' lives; we *can* work on our own reactions to them.

6. We believe that each person in our family—including ourselves—is entitled to a fair share of our time and resources.

7. We help each other consider alternatives, acknowledging that we can be more loving to our aging relatives when we are comfortable with our level of involvement in their care.

8. We summon courage to look at the reasons for any compulsive behavior that is giving us trouble; we do not base our decisions on the approval of others.

9. We admit that we cannot produce happiness for anyone else, including our aging loved ones; nor can we expect to fill all their needs.

10. We strive to clarify what is important to us and to consider any decisions on the basis of our true values, recognizing that any decision involves a cost.

11. We search for meaning in our experiences and seek to appreciate the benefits of knowing our relatives in their old age.

Workbook Contents

Scouting the Territory (Local Resources)

Collectively, you and the others in this seminar already know quite a bit about local resources. As you share experiences, jot down the names of contact persons and phone numbers. Make a note of who has used the service or knows about it.

Agencies for private nurses, LPN's, housekeepers, companions, etc.:

Adult Day Care Centers:

Alzheimer's Disease and Related Disorders Association:

Area Agency on Aging:

Beauticians who make house calls:

Clothing for the handicapped:

Dentists:

Emergency Response Systems:

Family Service Agency:

Geriatric Assessment Center:

Geriatric psychiatrists:

Hospice:

Hospital Social Service department:

Housing for seniors:

Information and Referral or Crisis Management Hotline:

Insurance agents knowledgeable about medical and long-term care insurance:

Lawyers familiar with durable power of attorney, conservatorship, and living wills:

Legal Aid:

Meals on Wheels, nutrition sites:

Mental Health Association:

Nursing homes:

Nursing or gerontology departments of colleges:

Personal care/boarding homes:

Private duty nurses:

Private geriatric care consultants:

Rehabilitation center:

Rental medical equipment:

Respite care:

Self-Help groups for chronic illnesses:

Senior centers:

"Sitters," paid or volunteer:

Social Security office:

Student nurses:

Telephone reassurance program:

Transportation services:

Visiting nurses:

My Responsibility Tree

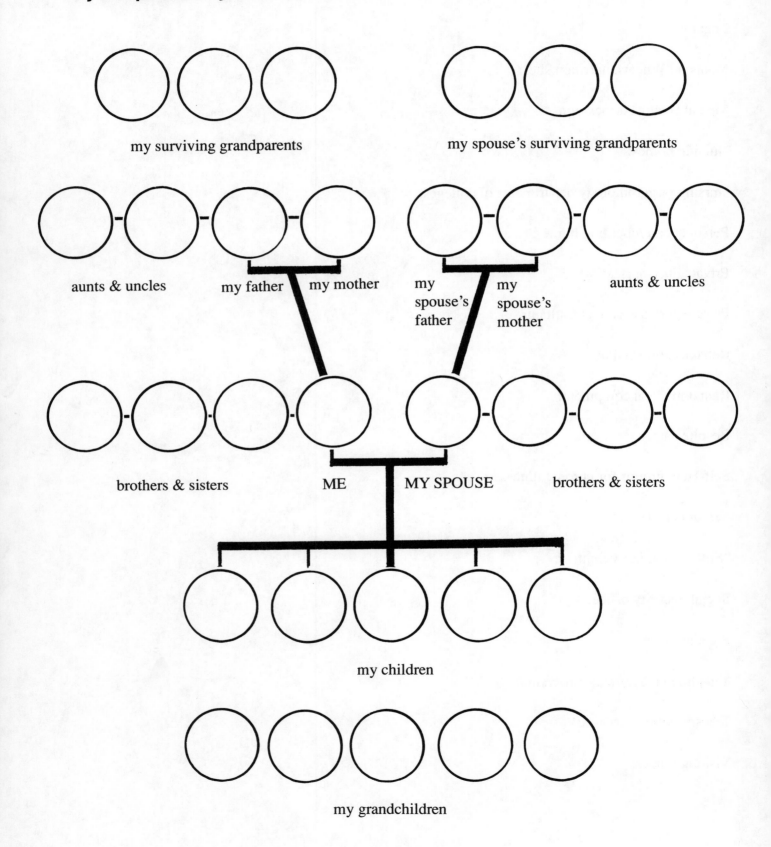

Guideposts for This Journey

1. Many things are going on in our lives, but in this group our relationship with elderly relatives is our primary concern.

2. The purpose of the group is to be helpful and supportive, not critical. As we are not wearing each other's shoes, so we will not judge how anyone else should walk.

3. All feelings—positive and negative—are acceptable. We make a special effort to become aware of and accept our *own* feelings.

4. We depend on confidentiality. We build trust by avoiding gossip. What we say here stays here.

5. Each of us will try to attend every meeting. In dire emergency, we'll let someone know ahead of time that we'll be absent.

6. We know that we have a lot to cover and pledge to cooperate in moving along in a timely way.

7. We expect to become a caring, sharing support network for each other.

Baggage (Feelings Expressed in Our Small Group)

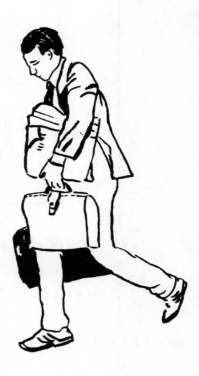

From Quicksand to Solid Ground (The Adjustment Process)

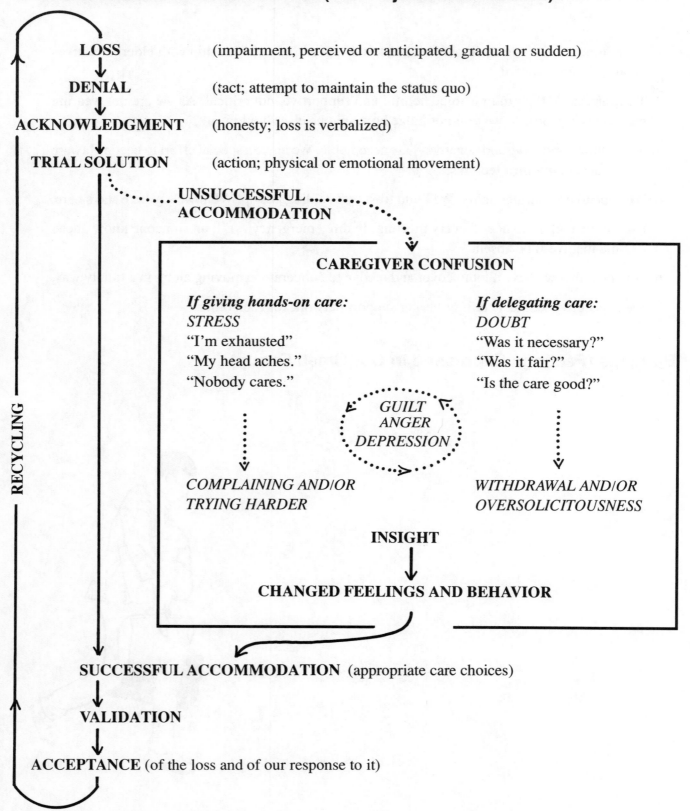

LOSS (impairment, perceived or anticipated, gradual or sudden)

DENIAL (tact; attempt to maintain the status quo)

ACKNOWLEDGMENT (honesty; loss is verbalized)

TRIAL SOLUTION (action; physical or emotional movement)

UNSUCCESSFUL ACCOMMODATION

CAREGIVER CONFUSION

If giving hands-on care:
STRESS
"I'm exhausted"
"My head aches."
"Nobody cares."

If delegating care:
DOUBT
"Was it necessary?"
"Was it fair?"
"Is the care good?"

GUILT ANGER DEPRESSION

COMPLAINING AND/OR TRYING HARDER

WITHDRAWAL AND/OR OVERSOLICITOUSNESS

INSIGHT

CHANGED FEELINGS AND BEHAVIOR

RECYCLING

SUCCESSFUL ACCOMMODATION (appropriate care choices)

VALIDATION

ACCEPTANCE (of the loss and of our response to it)

How Far Have I Come On the Journey?

LOSS

What physical losses has my relative sustained?

What mental losses?

What changes of housing, finances, or other circumstances?

What friends or family members have died or moved away?

How has my relationship with my relative changed?

What effect have these changes had on the rest of my life?

Have I had any of the following losses as a result of my relative's aging?

_____ I have less privacy.
_____ I have less time to spend with other people.
_____ I miss the old family home.
_____ I miss my former job.
_____ I miss the companionship my relative used to give me.
_____ I miss talking decisions over with my relative.
_____ I worry more about money.
_____ I hesitate to speak freely with other family members.
_____ I have given up my educational or travel plans.
_____ My present life seems boring.
_____ Thinking about my relative's impairments makes me sad.
_____ My physical health is suffering.
_____ I've quarreled with my brothers, sisters, or spouse.
_____ My relationship with my children is suffering.
_____ I don't have enough time for myself.
_____ I've almost lost my belief that I'm a loving person.

Other losses:

DENIAL

How have I tried to preserve the status quo—to keep things the same as always?

ACKNOWLEDGEMENT

Has something happened that forces me to face the reality of my relative's present impairments and/or future risk?

ACCOMMODATION

If I've tried a solution, what have I done?

In what ways is it working?

Has the solution caused any stress for me or others?

What doubts do I have about my solution?

Does my relative want me to do something else?

Does another family member want me to do anything differently?

Am *I* still searching for a better solution?

Do I sometimes feel like I am waiting for the other shoe to drop? What else?

Do you begin to understand why there are times you feel rotten? There seems to be no way to arrive at acceptance except through grief and pain—and often through doubt, guilt, stress, and anger as well. That's okay. Pain doesn't kill us.

If you are in this Seminar, you probably have not reached ACCEPTANCE yet. When you do, you can write your own last chapter.

Messages from Prior Travelers

Megan:

"I think for myself the most important factor was just being there in the group, and I'm not sure what this means. I'm very glad I came. My own problems are not so bad when I learn of some others."

Sally:

"When Anneta Kraus, Director of Geriatric Planning Services, a private consulting agency, visited our support group, we asked her, 'What do you do if your *relative* denies there has been any loss or change?' Anneta replied that about the only thing you can do—and it's hard—is withdraw support.

"She says if my Dad insists he can perfectly well stay in his own apartment, and I'm the one who's doing the cleaning, the shopping, the errands and the cooking—then I can stop providing maid service. She says it's painful to watch everything falling apart, but my Dad has to come to some acknowledgement, too. He has to have his chance to grieve. When he's ready, perhaps he and I can approach a trial solution together. After all, he is mentally competent; he deserves a voice in orchestrating his own lifestyle—just as I deserve to orchestrate mine.

"She says the more responsibility *he* takes for any decisions, the less regret *I'll* have."

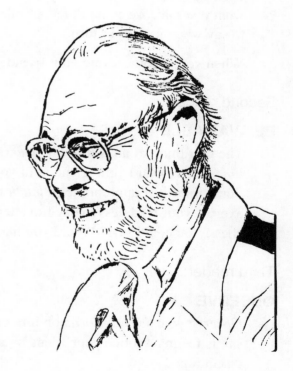

Chuck:

"I think maybe we can take too much control.

"I've been trying to persuade my mother to give up her car, and she's quite annoyed with me. Her room-mate told me that after my last visit Mom exploded, and finished by saying, '…and furthermore, the next time I get married, I'm *not* having any children!'"

Active Listening, the All-Weather Skill

First reader:

Active Listening is a counseling and friendship skill that reassures others you are "there" for them when they have a problem—that you accept them and are on their side. You cannot, of course, Actively Listen to someone with whom you are having an argument. As long as you are arguing you are not on that person's side! Only if you are willing and able to set your *own* feelings aside temporarily can you help your friend in this way.

At times we must honor our own feelings and cannot give this attention to another. That's okay, too. Once we possess the skill, we can *decide* when to use it.

The difference between Active Listening and an ordinary conversation is that here there is no exchange of views. While Actively Listening, you do not respond to statements with a statement of your own. Instead, you reflect thoughts back as accurately as possible, helping others become more aware of what they think and feel. As a first step, we practiced listening in today's opening exercise. As you spoke, your neighbor paid close attention in order to repeat exactly what you said. We couldn't let our minds wander or get all wrapped up in what *we* were going to say when it was our turn.

When you become aware your friend is troubled, begin with Active Listening.

Second reader:

BE AVAILABLE

The first thing to do is to *make yourself available physically. Find a quiet place and enough time.* Turn toward your friend until you are *face to face. Lean forward.* Establish *eye contact.* Sometimes it is appropriate to *touch* the other person sympathetically. Let your whole body express your readiness to pay full attention to whatever your friend wants to get off his or her chest. You could say: "Would you like to tell me about it?"

Third reader:

OBSERVE

Observe your friend. *Focus* on him or her and *resist distractions. Notice clues* to how he or she is feeling. Notice your friend's jaw…hands…voice…. You could say: "You look a little discouraged today."

Fourth reader:

LISTEN

Listen with your heart as well as your ears. *Think* about what life must be like for your friend right now. This person is doing the best he or she can in the situation. *Be non-judgmental.* Often all that is needed is to *wait quietly, nodding your head.* If your friend seems stuck, restate the last idea you heard in an encouraging way or utter a soft "Hmmm." Very skillful listeners are able to paraphrase without adding thoughts of their own, but it is safer for beginners to *repeat exactly* the last few words their friend said. You may think this will be too "obvious" or that you'll feel silly, but thoughts and feelings may not be apparent to either of you until you do this. Very likely your "technique" will be ignored as both of you concentrate on pinning down the problem. "Oh, so that's what's been bothering me!" It's better not to ask questions; questions might interrupt or guide the train of thought. Instead provide time for half-conscious concerns to rise into awareness. At this stage, listening is more helpful than making suggestions. *Avoid giving advice.* Jumping in to solve the problem will only frustrate your friend. You could say: "To you it seems as if…"

Fifth reader:

RESPOND

Echo and accept your friend's feelings. Listen with imagination. The actual words may be saying, "I didn't want to go to that picnic anyhow." But the sad face and tone of voice may be indicating disappointment. *Respond to what you perceive the feelings to be.* "You're feeling left out." Respond to the *situation*, too. "You're feeling left out because everyone else has plans for today and you don't." If you're wrong, your friend will tell you. "No, I was just thinking…" *Persevere.* Keep going until you have a good idea what the feelings are.

Sixth reader:

ACCEPT

Then *accept* them. You could say: "I can understand how you feel that way." Take your friend's problem and feelings seriously.

At this point most of us have to bite our tongues to keep from saying, "Why don't you go to the movies? Or invite Hank over? Or take Snoopy for a walk?" When a friend is in pain, we're hurting too, and we have a stake in feeling like Successful Helpers. Don't jump in with quick solutions! Listen! It's okay for people to have problems. They grow by handling them.

Distress Signals

Here are some sample "openers" that might tip you off to the presence of a problem. Which are the Active Listening responses?

1. Friend: "I don't know what to do. I'd love to apply for that teaching job that was advertised in **The Packet**—it's a wonderful opportunity—but Joe says a woman's place is in the home."

   __ (a) "Well, for heaven's sake, he ought to be glad you're willing to work; two paychecks!"

   __ (b) "That job really appeals to you, but you're uncertain about whether or not to apply.

   __ (c) "Well, I never thought a woman should go back to work until her kids are in junior high."

2. Friend: "My boss says if I won't work Friday nights he'll have to consider giving my job to someone else."

   __ (a) "You sound worried you might lose your job."

   __ (b) "That man makes me mad! It's time you looked for another position!"

   __ (c) "What's so bad about working Friday nights? You'd still have Saturday nights free."

3. Friend: "I went to the doctor today and he told me the results of some tests I took last week."

   __ (a) "You go to Dr. Benson, don't you. Is he any good?"

   __ (b) "Medicine can do wonderful things these days, but the bills are out of sight. It cost us $300 just for Jeannie's wisdom teeth."

   __ (c) "Do you want to talk about it?"

4. Friend: "It's getting so I hate to ride with Uncle Morris. He seems totally oblivious to the other traffic on the road. This morning he went right through a red light!"

   __ (a) "Really, the state police ought to retest everybody over eighty!"

   __ (b) "Well, just refuse to get in the car with him then."

   __ (c) "You're worried he might have an accident and hurt somebody, aren't you?"

Active Listening Checklist

Did I:	A Connie	B Alice	C	D	E
MAKE MYSELF AVAILABLE?					
Find a quiet place, enough time?	___	___	___	___	___
Sit face to face?	___	___	___	___	___
Lean forward?	___	___	___	___	___
Make eye contact?	___	___	___	___	___
Touch if appropriate?	___	___	___	___	___
OBSERVE?					
Focus on my friend?	___	___	___	___	___
Resist distractions?	___	___	___	___	___
Notice body language, tone of voice?	___	___	___	___	___
LISTEN?					
Remain non-judgmental?	___	___	___	___	___
Nod head? Wait quietly?	___	___	___	___	___
Repeat key words or ideas?	___	___	___	___	___
Avoid giving advice?	___	___	___	___	___
Avoid asking questions?	___	___	___	___	___
RESPOND?					
Respond to perceived feelings?	___	___	___	___	___
Respond to feelings *and* reasons?	___	___	___	___	___
Persevere?	___	___	___	___	___
ACCEPT?					
Confirm the reality of the problem?	___	___	___	___	___

Being accepted *where they are* enables people to go on to other steps of the problem-solving process.

Staying on Track

If you need someone to listen and your friend is pushing toward solutions, you can remind him or her of what you need. The following sentences may help:

"No, that's not what I said. What I said was…"

"Wait a minute. Let me think about that."

"I think you're giving me your opinion; what I said was…"

"It's not helpful to me right now to know what you did; I need more time to clarify my own thinking. I said…"

"You're problem-solving. I'm not ready for that yet. I was trying to remember…"

"I seem to be saying, 'Yes, but,' a lot. I think we must be problem-solving. Let's go back. What I was saying was…"

"Whoa. You're getting ahead of me. I still haven't figured out how I really feel about this whole situation."

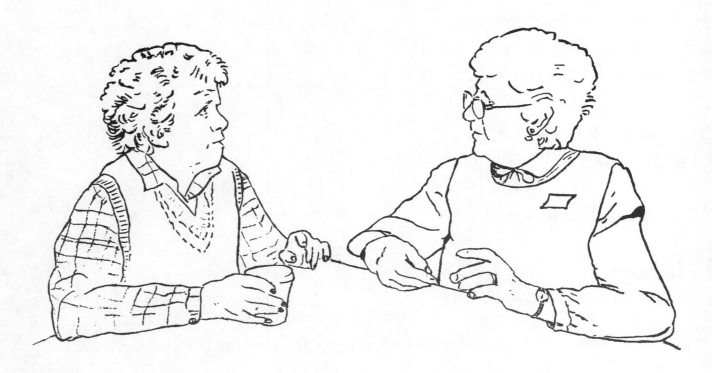

Eavesdropping (Skit)

Possible "props": scissors, flowers, vase, cup of coffee, spoon.

Narrator: Scene I. Sue is sitting at her neighbor Connie's kitchen table stirring her coffee. Connie is arranging flowers at the sink, when Sue says…

Sue: I just don't know what I'm going to do with Mona. (sigh) I'm at my wit's end!

Connie: (leaves the sink and sits down opposite Sue; leans her elbows on the table and looks at her.) What's the matter, Sue? Do you want to talk about it?

Sue: Mrs. Robinson called me yesterday complaining about how many times Mona's been late to school. I didn't know what to say.

Connie: Oh, boy. Embarrassing, huh.

Sue: It sure was. After all, I don't sleep late in the mornings and let the kids fend for themselves. Connie, you know I'm always up at 6:15 and cook a good hot breakfast.

Connie: Yes, I know. You feel like you're doing your part to get Mona off on the right foot.

Sue: I sure do! It makes me so mad that she dawdles away the time after breakfast until we all have to rush around like crazy looking for her homework…*and* her umbrella…*and* her lunch money…*and* her permission slip—all the stuff she should have organized the night before.

Connie: It really bugs you, doesn't it, that Mona is so disorganized.

Sue: Right! I hate to have to jump up from the table and rush around, just to get her out the door.

Connie: When you're enjoying your breakfast you hate to jump up.

Sue: I sure do! For heaven's sake, what kind of mood do you think that puts *me* in for the day? I'm really frustrated about it!

Connie: (nods her head and waits)

Sue: It seems like there's just nothing I can do to make Mona prompt. I've nagged and I've scolded and we've taken away her TV privileges too…and nothing seems to work.

Connie: (continues nodding her head)

Sue: It's like she's deliberately doing it, just to show we can't boss her around!

Connie: You feel like Mona is dawdling on purpose. You're frustrated because you really have no control over *when* she gets to school.

Sue: Hey. I think maybe you just put your finger on what's bothering me. I am losing control, aren't I?

Connie: It sure looks like it. Hard to get used to, isn't it, Sue?

Sue: Oh, well… (sighs again) I guess I'll survive the teens somehow. Everybody else does. Thanks for helping me, Connie.

Narrator: Sue thanked Connie for helping her, and Connie *was* a help, though she didn't make a single suggestion about getting Mona to school. Let's thank our actors with a round of applause.

🌸 🌸 🌸

Narrator: And now for Scene II. Sue has another neighbor, Alice. Sue is sitting at Alice's kitchen table stirring her coffee. Alice is arranging flowers at the sink, when Sue says…

Sue: I just don't know what I'm going to do with Mona. (sigh) I'm at my wit's end!

Alice: (continues arranging flowers and says, over her shoulder) Well, what's God's gift to the tenth grade done now? Tie up the telephone all night?

Sue: No. Mrs. Robinson called me yesterday complaining about how many times Mona's been late to school, and I didn't know what to say.

Alice: For heaven's sake, Sue, you're not going to let Old Lady Robinson upset you! She's been at that school since the year one!

Sue: Well, maybe so, but she really put me on the spot. I get so mad at Mona (when she)…

Alice: (interrupting) Oh, lay off the kid, can't you, Sue? You're too strict with her.

Sue: Too strict?! What do you mean? (defensively) You have to be strict with girls. And Mona's so mature for her age…

Alice: Oh, really, Sue. If you'd permit her to wear eye makeup to school, she wouldn't have to sneak it into her notebook and spend half the first period in the girls' room, putting it on. Oh, dear…now where did I put those scissors?

Sue: That's easy for you to say; you've got all boys. Girls are a lot harder to bring up.

Alice: (airily) Oh, You worry too much, Honey. Relax! The kids are only young once. Didn't you ever want to have a little fun when you were Mona's age?

Sue: (doubtfully) I suppose so…but my mother wouldn't ever let me…and *she* thinks I give Mona too much freedom as it is. Oh, Alice, (big sigh) why can't I manage better?

Practice Makes For Progress

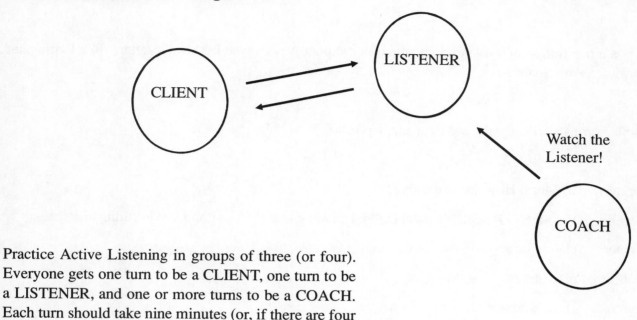

Practice Active Listening in groups of three (or four). Everyone gets one turn to be a CLIENT, one turn to be a LISTENER, and one or more turns to be a COACH. Each turn should take nine minutes (or, if there are four in the group, six or seven minutes).

CLIENT: Talk about a problem from daily life, one that has nothing to do with aging. Try to think of a real problem, like a hassle with your kids, your job, the neighbor's pet, or the auto mechanic.

LISTENER: Practice Active Listening. You may consult the checklist before you begin. When you are stopped after four minutes, ask the Coach for feedback. "Was I leaning forward?" "Was I repeating key words or ideas?" "Anything else?"

COACH(ES): Watch the *Listener*, not the Client. Do not try to help solve the problem! Do not say anything. (You are permitted to point to a phrase on the checklist.) Your task is to watch the "actors" closely and observe the extent to which the Listener is listening correctly. After four minutes (use a watch or timer), stop the practice. Give the Listener one minute to ask for feedback.

Please don't be shy about making suggestions. This skill is difficult at first, and it's no favor to let your friend practice incorrectly. You'll have your turn to receive help, too.

Allow the listening to resume and continue for the remainer of that turn, during which the Listener practices with your suggestions in mind.

As each Listener finishes, take a minute to help him or her fill out column C of the checklist. Give a plus (+) for every part of the skill the Listener remembered at least once.

Visiting Mama (Re-enactment of a Class Exercise)

This is a transcription of a role play in which Participant A portrayed her own mother while Participant B portrayed Participant A.

Possible "props": wheelchair, walker, cane, lap robe.

Daughter: Hi, Mom. How are you today?

Mother: (Woodenly) Hello… (softer) Hello. I'm not good. I'm not good…everything hurts me.

Daughter: (Gently, practicing Active Listening) Oh…Mama… You've got pains.

Mother: Yes… Everything. Sure…

Daughter: Oh… Your arms…

Mother: Everything hurts.

Daughter: And your head…

Mother: Go away. Don't touch me. I'm mad at you.

Daughter: You're mad at me today.

Mother: You put me in a place like this. I…I don't want to be here. I don't like it here. I want to go home.

Daughter: You really want to come home, don't you?

Mother: Sure.

Daughter: You don't like it here.

Mother: No. I don't like it here. I yell and yell and scream and nobody hears me. Nobody ever listens to me. Nobody comes. I have to wait very long.

Daughter: Aaaaah… You wait too long for them to come and take care of you.

Mother: How do you…How do you feel today?

Daughter: Well, I'm pretty good today.

Mother: Yeah. That's good. How are the children?

Daughter: Oh, they're fine. You know, Johnny's getting ready for his graduation.

Mother: Yeah, I know… I…I have a pain in my chest. I can't breathe too good.

Daughter: Something's wrong with your breathing today.

Mother: Yeah. I think I have to die.

Daughter: Oh, Mama! You're thinking about dying.

Mother: Sure. It's time. I think it's time.

Daughter: You're so tired.

Mother: Sure.

Daughter: You're really tired. It's been a long time, hasn't it?

Mother: Yeah. Yeah, but…but I don't like it here.

Daughter: I know. You really aren't happy here.

Mother: Nooo. It's your fault. It's your fault.

Daughter: (long audible sigh) Oh, Mama…I love you anyway!

Mother: I love you too, but… (beginning to cry) I don't like it here. (sobs)

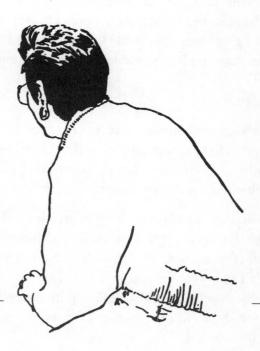

Expressing Love to the Elderly

First reader:

Given enough money, it would be possible to hire somebody to do almost anything for our relatives. Almost, but not quite. Nobody else can be *us* for them. Nobody else can give them *our* love and *our* support.

In the nature of things, old people sustain many losses. Our elderly relatives may have lost jobs, homes, spouses, friends, even their health. They are going to feel sad some of the time—maybe most of the time. If we allow ourselves to empathize with their feelings, it can be pretty painful, especially if we believe we ought to make them happy.

On the other hand, if we avoid hearing their feelings, who else in the world can they count on to understand and care?

Second reader:

To Listen Actively to our relatives in their sadness, it is necessary to overcome our own pain and discomfort. When Bea visits her mother in the nursing home and her mother says, "Take me home. I want to go home!" Bea's impulse is to reply out of her own defensiveness, "Now, Mama, you know the doctor says you need to be here. Besides, I can't take proper care of you at home. I can't even lift you."

Do you think for one minute Bea's mother is going to reply, "Oh, yeah, that's right. I am bedridden and incontinent, aren't I?" Not on your tintype! She's an old lady, sick, and living among strangers. She feels life has stopped. She feels unloved and worthless. She doesn't *want* to understand Bea's problems with the situation. She wants Bea to understand *hers*.

Third reader:

Bea's temptation was to respond out of her own exasperation. But her mother needed Bea to respond to *her* feelings. An Active Listening response to "I want to go home," might be, "You really want to come home, don't you? I know." At least there's no temptation for Bea to problem-solve for her mother. There really isn't any solution.

What, then, can Bea do to comfort her mother? Probably the most important thing is just to *be there* for her. It would be easier for Bea to distract herself by talking to her mother's room-mate, fussing with the flowers, or having a conversation with the nursing assistant—anything rather than paying attention to her mother's pain. But Bea's full attention is what her mother needs, especially when she's feeling scared and cranky. When Bea takes her hand, looks her in the eye, and repeats word for word, her mother knows she's been heard; she's *sure* Bea *understands*.

Fourth reader:

Physical affection is another gift Bea can offer. As the other senses dim, touching becomes more important to old people. Even in families who have not before been particularly demonstrative, hugging, kissing, and hand-holding can become immensely valuable means of showing love to the elderly. If touching is not in your relative's present range of behavior, you will have to be the one to initiate it. You may be rebuffed a few times. Hang in there! Almost all older people come to appreciate love expressed through physical contact. When you sit facing your relative and take her hand, it helps her focus on you. You may even find, to your surprise, that she covers your hand with her other one and hangs on for dear life! People *need* affectionate touching; it's emotional vitamins. Don't you, yourself, love to hug a sleepy baby? Remember that old people may have lost other relationships that used to meet this need.

Fifth reader:

If this is a new idea to you and your relative, you might want to begin by brushing your aunt's hair or offering your dad an arm when walking together. Older persons who ambulate perfectly well enjoy the excuse to take an arm or hold your hand. It comforts them that, for the moment at least, they've really "got" you.

You, on the other hand, may find the feeling of "being got" unbearable. When we are under severe emotional pressure from our relative, we can't *stand* being clutched. We're feeling too clutched already! If this is the case, experiment with a shoulder or foot rub. You'll be in control and able to back away when you want to.

We're not telling you you *have* to touch your elderly relative. The last thing we want to do is lay another burden on you. Maybe you just don't have the inner resources right now to respond to that need. As you continue working through these lessons, and as you begin to regain control of your life, we hope you'll experiment with touching as a very effective way of showing love to your relative.

Sixth reader:

You may be touching your relative often during the normal course of the day's care. That's fine. Just remember that *functional* touching is not always interpreted as a symbol of emotional warmth. Find time for the touch that says, "I want to be right here, with you, right now." If the ill person is your spouse, it's especially important to provide chances for him or her to hug and kiss you back!

When Dorothy Died (Re-enactment of a Real-life Conversation)

This conversation took place in a nursing home where Jane was visiting a dear elderly friend. She had brought along a tape recorder and asked him to talk about what life was like for him. How quickly Active Listening takes one down into the heart of things!

Papa: Well, I miss my wife so much. Dear Dorothy! She was a wonderful woman.

Jane: Mm-hmmmm…yeah. It's been kinda lonesome with her gone, hasn't it?

Papa: Oh, yes. (slower) Yes. (still slower) Yes. But I'm glad she didn't have to suffer any longer in the condition she was in…at the time. She…she died on New Year's Eve and that was the time when we had that…well, all over the country, that flu or virus epidemic. And we were quarantined here, and I had…

Jane: You were sick, weren't you?

Papa: Yes, about three weeks, two weeks anyway, and I was in bed. I couldn't go to see her at the last…

Jane: Oh.

Papa: And…

Jane: That was too bad.

Papa: I never saw her after…even after she died. So…

Jane: You never got your chance to really say goodbye.

Papa: No…no.

Jane: Mm-hmmmm.

Papa: I had been going to see her three times a day…and…always, in the evening, she liked me to rub her forehead. Once she said, "I'm sure that even when I was dying I would recognize your hand on my forehead, and…

Jane: Oh…

Papa: I never had a chance.

Jane: Your hand wasn't able to be there.

Papa: No…no.

More Messages Along the Trail

Joanne:

"It turns out that Active Listening is a wonderful way to get along better with your spouse, your kids, your taxi driver, your boss—even yourself. Yes, I find out what *I* am feeling when I write in my Journal and read what I say!

"I feel more secure in the world now that I know Active Listening. I'll never have to be lonely and isolated again. Even when I'm an old lady, I'll be able to connect with somebody."

Eva:

"I've been delivering Meals on Wheels. Once a month, instead of taking the meals to people's homes, they bring the elderly together for a 'birthday dinner'. Last month, as I was helping Mrs. Jackson into the building, she said, 'You know me well enough to call me Jean.'

"'Well,' I replied, 'in that case I know you well enough to do this,' and gave her a big hug.

"To my dismay, Jean Jackson began to cry. The tears ran down her cheeks.

"'Oh. I'm sorry; I didn't mean to hurt you.'"

"'Oh, no, my dear. You didn't hurt me. But that's the first hug I've had since my husband died four years ago.'"

Warren:

"Although it seems simple (you only have to recognize problems, not solve them), Active Listening isn't easy. It's hard work for me to submerge my own views and care completely about another's.

"Nobody can be expected to Actively Listen to every problem anyone else has! It's a skill that's available when I have the time, the energy, and the desire to help. I have every right to chose whether and when to make that gift to someone."

Stella:

"I finally got up the nerve to touch my mother. She didn't seem to respond at all. But it felt awfully good to *me*."

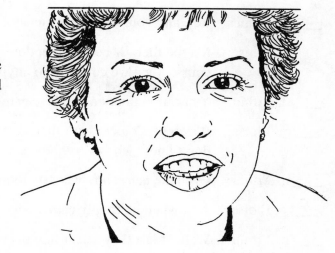

The Enjoyment of Misery

Here's a conversation you might overhear while waiting for the curtain to rise on **Hello, Dolly!** Obviously, nobody enjoys complaining more than Arthur and Eloise. Read (or listen to) the entire conversation once. Then go back and write a 1 in front of each sentence that complains about a problem nobody can do anything about. Write a 2 in front of each sentence that describes a problem somebody could change, but not the speaker. Write a 3 in front of each sentence describing a problem in which the speaker has some chance of influencing a change for the better.

_____ a. Eloise: Did you see that it's going to be a particularly cold winter?

_____ b. Arthur: Everybody ought to insulate their houses with this shredded-paper stuff. But they haven't, and they probably won't.

_____ c. Eloise: The trouble with people is, they never believe the scientists. They didn't protect their trees from the gypsy moths, either.

_____ d. Arthur: I never saw the gypsy moths so bad. I'll bet some of the trees won't make it through the winter.

_____ e. Eloise: That place the azalea died looks awful.

_____ f. Arthur: By the way, did I tell you Harry's invited himself for the holidays?

_____ g. Eloise: What?! The guest room is full of my sewing for the bazaar.

_____ h. Arthur: Well, you'll just have to move it. Harry never asks; he _tells_ you.

_____ i. Eloise: Honestly, Arthur, you make me so mad! Why don't you ever stand up to your brother? You've let him push you around for forty years.

_____ j. Arthur: Yes, and you've nagged me about it for the last twenty.

_____ k. Eloise: Maybe there'll be a tremendous snowstorm and he won't be able to get through. Of course, then we couldn't go anyplace, either.

_____ l. Arthur: You can't count on it. The weather always seems to do the opposite of what I want.

_____ m. Eloise: It's eight o'clock. Isn't that supposed to be curtain time? People are still coming in. I don't know why everybody can't be on time like us.

_____ n. Arthur: Even the paper boy was late tonight.

_____ o. Eloise: And when he finally came, what were the headlines? Earthquakes, floods, tornados!

_____ p. Arthur: Well, at last they're starting the overture. Darn! Now I'm thirsty.

Diagnosis

First reader:

Complaining certainly does pass the time, doesn't it? And if folks complain about situations they can't do anything about, they're saved from making any extra effort, too.

Eloise can't do anything about the cold winter (Type 1) or people's not believing the scientists (Type 2). She hasn't been able to get Arthur to stand up to his brother (Type 2), and she's been working on that one twenty years! She can't control a snowstorm (Type 1), nor can she make the theatre curtain rise (Type 2). As for the earthquakes, floods, and tornadoes (Type 1), forget it! Eloise *can* do some planting in the yard (Type 3). She can move her bazaar sewing, too, or let Harry sleep on the sofa (Type 3).

Second reader:

Arthur has managed to have this whole conversation without committing himself to a single constructive action. He can't make people insulate their houses (Type 2). He can't control the gypsy moths (Type 1). He thinks he can't tell Harry not to come (actually, probably a Type 3, but Arthur maintains it's a Type 2). He can't get Eloise to stop nagging him about Harry (Type 2). The weather always does the opposite of what he wants (Type 1) and the paper boy was late (Type 2). Arthur does not think of himself as an ineffective person; he is the much-put-upon victim of an unfeeling world. He didn't even get himself a drink of water! Arthur's sense of the world's being out of control comes at least partly from his failure to figure out what *he* could do to improve it.

Third reader:

Does anyone you know play "Ain't it awful?"

Families of the aging can get into a similar bind. Our lives can be complex and discouraging; we can feel like we can't *move*. That's when we need each other. We can help each other recognize the *parts* of our situations where we can act. If we could *not* do even one small thing to improve our lives, we would indeed be helpless. We would have no hope that things could ever be better. But we are not helpless. There's always something we can do about our part of a situation. In the next few weeks, we'll begin to renew our control.

Can Anything Be Done?

1. After supper Billy Sheddar rides over to Kevin's house so they can work on homework together but he often forgets his bike light. Mrs. Sheddar is afraid Billy may have an accident when he rides home after dark. What kind of problem is Billy's forgetfulness for his mother?

    ____ Type 1. Nobody can do anything about it.
    ____ Type 2. Somebody can do something about it, but not Mrs. Sheddar.
    ____ Type 3. There is at least one action Mrs. Sheddar could take.

2. Kate's friend, Erma, has terrible fights with her mother, who nags and nit-picks until finally Erma blows up at her. Kate finds these scenes embarrassing and sometimes get caught in the crossfire. What kind of problem is the situation for Kate?

    ____ Type 1. Nobody can do anything about it.
    ____ Type 2. Somebody can do something about it, but not Kate.
    ____ Type 3. There is something Kate can do.

3. Last week the beautiful old tree in Jack Hill's front yard was struck by lightning and split down the middle. Jack feels sick about it. Jack was looking forward to putting up a swing for his grandchildren. What kind of problem is the splintered tree for Jack?

    ____ Type 1. Nobody can do anything about it.
    ____ Type 2. Somebody can do something about it, but not Jack.
    ____ Type 3. There is one thing Jack can do to save his tree.

4. Sharon and Michael's baby was born with a hip deformity. Sharon just can't get over a terrible feeling of guilt. Michael tries to tell her he loves little Cory and everything's going to be all right. Sharon just can't believe him. What kind of problem is Cory's hip for Sharon?

    ____ Type 1. Nobody can do anything about it for now.
    ____ Type 2. Somebody can do something about it, but not Sharon.
    ____ Type 3. Sharon should "snap out of it."

5. Bella's husband, Ron, hardly finishes a meal before he lights a cigarette. Ron's father died—very painfully—from emphysema. Bella had hoped it would motivate Ron to stop smoking, but it hasn't. Every time Bella broaches the subject, Ron snaps at her. Is Ron's smoking more than one kind of problem for Bella?

    ____ Type 1. Nobody can make Ron quit smoking.
    ____ Type 2. Somebody might be able to terminate Ron's smoking habit, but not Bella.
    ____ Type 3. Bella can minimize the consequences of Ron's habit *for herself.*

Mud, Flood, and Blood (Skit)

Possible "prop": umbrella

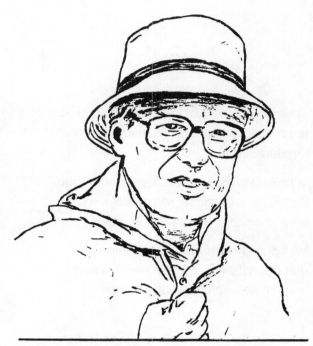

Steve: (coming in soaking wet) Wow! Is the rain ever coming down! Do you ever get water in the basement? The ground is still frozen, and it's pouring.

Barbara: Do we get water! Last spring we had to call the fire department twice to pump us out. The water got so deep it ruined the motor on the freezer, and I felt sick about it. I had to give or throw away quite a bit of food.

Steve: Must have made a mess, too. Didn't Ben do anything?

Barbara: What can you do when the water is actually gushing up through the floor? Stop the rain? You know, we thought if the builder would just finish grading next door, it would solve the drainage problem for the whole neighborhood, but, of course, the house hasn't sold. Everybody's complaining about the mess.

Steve: Couldn't you get the contractor to do something?

Barbara: Ben tried, but all we got was a big runaround. It makes me mad. Ben said he felt like marching over there and giving him a bloody nose! Probably with the housing market so slow he just doesn't want to spend the money.

Steve: Well, you can't sit here and declare a flood emergency every time we get a spring rain.

Barbara: Right! That's why we finally went ahead and installed a sump pump. We put off spending the money, but—believe me—the peace of mind is worth it! Every time I hear that motor go on downstairs, it gives me such a comfortable, protected feeling. Listen, there it goes now. It's noisy…and I love it.

Classifying Caregiving Problems

Write a 1 in front of each statement that describes a problem *nobody* can do anything about.

Write a 2 in front of each statement that describes a problem *somebody* may be able to rectify, but not the speaker.

Write a 3 in front of each statement that describes a problem *the speaker* may be able to confront successfully.

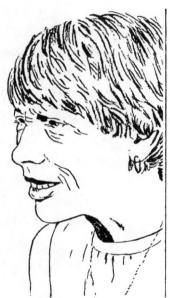

_____ a. "My mother doesn't like the nursing home."

_____ b. "My sisters won't help; we should all take turns."

_____ c. "Everybody chips in to pay Dad's companion except my cheapskate brother-in-law; he absolutely refuses."

_____ d. "Dad can't control his bladder any more."

_____ e. "The nursing home aides don't always come as soon as my husband calls."

_____ f. "Mom blames me when she can't remember where she put something."

_____ g. "My aunt insists on staying in her apartment, even though there have been three muggings in her neighborhood."

_____ h. "I really don't like spending every Sunday with my in-laws."

My Six-Square Grid

PROBLEM SITUATIONS	NEGATIVE FEELINGS

A	Type 1 Elements Nobody Can Change	B
C	Type 2 Elements Somebody Else Can Change, But Not Me	D
E	Type 3 Elements I Can Change	F

Getting a Handle on Aggravation

First. Write a statement describing someone's behavior that "bugs" you.

Second. If you haven't already included this information, add an explanation indicating why the behavior annoys you. Why should *you* care?

Third. If you haven't already included this information, add a description of how you feel about the annoying behavior and how you react to it. Draw one line under the words that describe your <u>feelings</u>. Draw a <u>double line</u> under the words that describe how you react.

Fourth. Now it's only necessary to discover what you may be doing—or neglecting to do—that permits this situation to continue. We're looking for enabling behavior, and the word "behavior" means that our body does (or doesn't do) something.

What do you do with your hands...your feet...your mouth...that permits the annoying behavior to continue? Or...What do you avoid doing?

If you have found something that you are doing that you have the power to change (if you wish to) write it in Square E on page 31.

Just Dreaming….

Most seminar participants discover they are doing some things they don't really want to be doing, but that they can't stop. There seems to be no rescue and no escape. Just for once, don't be practical. Let yourself dream a little. Who knows? Some dreams come true.

Complete any sentence that jogs your mind. This is a private page, just for you; you will not be asked to share what you write.

It would be heavenly if I could

If only I had the nerve to

If I didn't feel so responsible, I would

To tell the truth, what I really want to do is

Sometimes I wish I could just say to my elderly relative, "

I wish I could tell my sister (or brother)

I wish I could stop

I wish I didn't keep trying to

I wish I didn't allow

Footprints

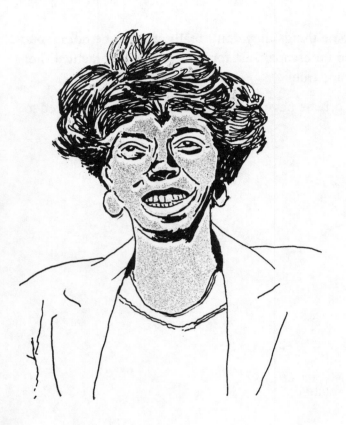

Melissa:

"My mother was very sick; she hadn't been out of her bedroom for a couple of years. My one sister and I were wearing ourselves out taking care of her. In fact, my husband said, 'You might as well move over to your mother's; you're there all the time.'

"My problem was that my other sisters wouldn't help. I tried and tried talking to them, but they just got mad at me. If we had just all taken turns, we could have done it. But they refused. I thought they were being really bad daughters.

"I was going crazy. My sisters weren't speaking to me. My husband was mad at me. I felt like I was being pulled in a dozen different directions.

"The first couple of meetings of the seminar, I was in tears. Then one day it dawned on me. I was trying to do something that couldn't be done. My sisters were *never* going to agree to my plan.

"Once I realized that, I was free to make other arrangements, and I did."

Lynn:

"The thought of deliberately identifying my own responsibility in a problem situation makes me feel both free and frightened. Free, because it means I have the *power* to begin getting unstuck. Frightened, because it also means I'll have to accept the consequences of using that power. If I'm not a passive victim, then my decisions and actions have significance, for my own life and the lives of others. That's a sobering thought. On the whole, I think I like it."

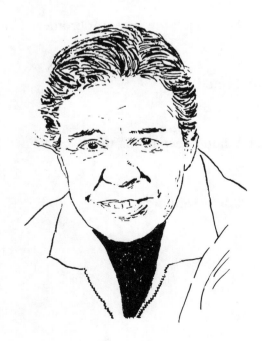

Finding My Way (Interview)

Partners are to take turns interviewing each other. When you are the CLIENT, hand your workbook to the INTERVIEWER, who will ask questions, listen, and jot down his or her observations about your situation. When you are the interviewer, don't solve problems. Just *listen* and get it down in writing.

Interview Questions

What is the WORST THING about your present situation? [Use Active Listening.]

Is this WORST THING a Type 1, Type 2, or Type 3 element? [Circle one.]

Have you been trying to do something that is impossible?

Have you been permitting someone to do something that irritates you?

What would be the BEST THING that could happen in your situation?

Do you have the power to make the BEST THING happen? Why or why not?

There are one or two things that, if you could do them, would make an immediate improvement in the quality of your life. What are they?

[If your partner can't think of a single thing, just say, "Well, maybe something will occur to you during the week." You will have an opportunity to offer suggestions in Session 5.]

Pinpointing a Destination

Our part in perpetuating our own problems is often more apparent to someone else than to us. That's why we can be so helpful to each other. You should be holding your partner's workbook. Consult with your partner and fill in the blanks of at least one *specific, measurable, attainable* objective for him or her. When determining objectives, it's not necessary to "Win the War." Identifying skirmishes in which there is a good chance of success is just as helpful.

If you can come up with more than one objective, all the better. You and your partner will then have a choice of what to work on together next week.

ACHIEVABLE OBJECTIVES

_____ (*Partner's name*) feels _____ (*negative feeling*)

because he or she is _____ (*an action verb—something he or she is doing …or trying in vain to do…or permitting…or avoiding doing…or failing to utilize.*)

and he or she wants _____ (*objective—something he or she wants to do or feel differently*).

_____ (*Partner's name*) feels _____ (*negative feeling*)

because he or she is _____ (*an action verb—something he or she is doing …or trying in vain to do…or permitting…or avoiding doing…or failing to utilize.*)

and he or she wants _____ (*objective—something he or she wants to do or feel differently*).

Jane's Story (Monologue)

When I came to Carol's seminar, my stomach had been hurting for weeks. We had invited my mother-in-law to live with us and I knew I ought to love her—I thought I did love her—but my body was telling me something was wrong.

When we came to this part of the seminar, I decided to tackle one small element of my problem, as Carol suggested. "I feel jumpy because I cannot seem to relax and go on about my life when Nana is in the house; I want to feel not pestered by Nana."

This was a very difficult assignment. I was asking myself to change my *feelings*. From deep inside I seemed to hear, "I'll be darned if I will; I have a right to my own feelings, at least! I was not born for this!"

I would have done better to work on the troublesome behavior that my feelings produced. A better problem statement would have been: "I feel frustrated because I am not going on about my life, and I want to get down to business." Stated that way, I might have been able to get out of the box. Many households *have* managed to successfully integrate an aging parent.

As it happened, things took a different turn. I became aware of a more inclusive objective: "I feel angry because we are permitting Nana to live with us and I want to move her out of my house." Suddenly I was very clear about the goal. My problem was that I could imagine only one honorable reason for moving her; the move would be legitimate only if she went to the hospital—or died. And, at age 87, she was rousingly healthy!

When Nana first came, a woman in our church—a woman with impeccable credentials, as she had *both* her mother *and* her mother-in-law living with her—said to me, "Yes, my dear, I know it's hard, but you're doing the *right thing*." For months her comments echoed in my mind. If bringing Nana was "the right thing," how could I ever send her away and declare myself "wrong?" Thus does a neighbor's judgment, even a complimentary judgment, destroy our freedom.

Freedom! Just to get out of the house, by myself, became a weekly treat. And guess what I did! I spent those few precious hours visiting nursing homes! But I didn't locate any that would be right for a disoriented, conversational, physically vigorous woman.

It wasn't appropriate for Nana to live with us, but neither was it appropriate for her to live in a nursing home with sick people. She was betwixt and between, and didn't belong anywhere. That was the first problem.

The second problem was that I couldn't let go.

Why Was Jane Stuck?

If Jane had been telling you her troubles, she would have used these sentences. They all describe something Jane herself was doing (Type 3 problems). Theoretically, Jane could have changed her own behavior. Why didn't she?

After listening to Jane's complaints, perhaps you would have been able to guess what Whispers she was hearing in her head. Mark an X before each unspoken thought you sense may have been keeping her "in a box." Note: one problem may arise from several sources.

1. "I hate answering the same question twenty times, dragging Nana along on errands, and watching uninteresting TV shows!"

   ____ "But she keeps asking for attention."
   ____ "After all, I'm responsible for making her happy."
   ____ "I feel guilty. We uprooted her and dismantled her house."

2. "I'm making myself available to Nana's confused mind night and day."

   ____ "She just can't organize herself and rattles around the house."
   ____ "It's impolite not to respond when I'm spoken to."
   ____ "If I'm extra, extra good to Nana, maybe she'll love me as a real person again."

3. "I really don't want Nana to live with us; why are we keeping her here?"

   ____ "There doesn't seem to be any other good place for her to live."
   ____ "If Nana doesn't live with us, it means we don't love her."
   ____ "If I don't take care of Nana, maybe my kids won't take care of me when I'm old."

P.S. from Jane: Perhaps you'd like to know what happened next. We realized I had to have some time off. I found a board-and-care home out in the country that would accept Nana as a "day student." Three or four times a week Mark would drive her out on his way to work; I'd pick her up in the afternoon. At first she went "kicking and screaming," but Mark would insist. It felt bad to force her, but we did. And when spring came, Nana began to appreciate the beauty of "That Place." When she got bored, she'd even ask to be driven out there! Eventually we got the courage to leave her overnight, and the roof didn't cave in! So, when I finally had the nerve to ask, "How would you feel about not living with us?" she said, "Well, I'm already acquainted at That Place; I could move there."

I said, "How about Monday?!"

We paid another resident to look after her. Josephine did a wonderful job. She had nothing else to do! She washed Nana and combed her hair, saw that she got to meals on time, took her for little walks, and located her purse when the ice cream truck came. She tucked Nana in with a kiss at night. She always had Nana dressed up and ready when we arrived to take her to church or home for a meal. There were still "poor me" phone calls, of course, but on the whole we all adjusted pretty well.

Nana had plenty of company all day long, and I had blessed quiet. We both learned that her living elsewhere didn't mean we didn't love her. What a relief to hug and kiss her again and mean it!

The Clash of Forces—Jane's Battle Line

Freeing Forces → **POW!** ← **Imprisoning Forces**

BATTLE LINE (tension, stress, pressure)

OBJECTIVE

Freeing Forces	Imprisoning Forces
My husband cares.	Lack of facilities.
I'm getting good advice.	Lack of time to look.
Seminar friends encourage me.	Mrs. Lamb says I'm doing the right thing.
My children understand.	I feel guilty.
I'm eager for a better life.	Nana's resistance.
Nana has enough money.	"I should make her happy."
	I want our old relationship back again!
	Aren't I a loving person?

Reflections

My aging relative needs…
It's just not practical for my relative to…
I haven't been able to find…
One resource I sure wish I had is…
These days I never seem to have enough…
I've been taught I should always…
The quotation my head keeps repeating is…
I believe a "good daughter" or a "good son" ought to…
I'm terribly sorry that I…
I feel guilty that I don't really want…
By myself I can't…
I am afraid of…
It makes me furious when…
I've been hurt too often by…
If I defy my parent…
It's ungrateful to…
I really need…
I wish I had never promised…
It doesn't seem fair that I'm so healthy and…
Everybody in the family acts like they expect…
Ever since I was small, I always…
I would feel ashamed if…
In my heart, I am comparing myself to…
I think I know what my relative wants from me; what I want from him or her is…
I'm longing for…
I pray for the courage to try…
My religious tradition teaches me that…
When my relative scolds me, I feel like…
Maybe I haven't been good enough to deserve…
My relative always wanted to control my life, and I always…
Part of me is not willing to share the care of my parent with…
If I didn't have this problem with my aging relative, I would…
I would feel neglectful if I didn't…
One mistake I never want to make is…
The person whose good opinion I most cherish is…
I always expected that…

Reactions

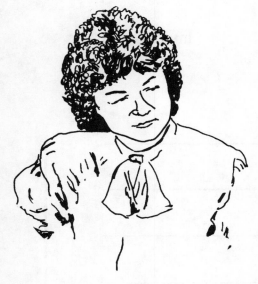

How did the Guided Meditation feel to you?

Did you enjoy relaxing?

Did the five minutes of silence seem long or short to you?

Do you feel a little more in touch with an inward part of yourself?

Is there any insight you'd like to share?

Anything else?

Freedom

Someone once said, "It's not the things we don't know that get us into trouble; it's the things we *do* know that ain't so!"

Our feelings are something over which, believe it or not, we have some control. We can change what we are thinking or believing that causes the feelings. But first we have to recognize it.

Perhaps we have discovered some thoughts or beliefs that are making us do things in a way that is causing problems. Today we might want to reflect on how important those beliefs or expectations are to us and whether or not we want to spend the rest of our lives with them. It would be all right if we'd decide just to let some of them go.

The Clash of Forces—My Battle Line

Freeing Forces

POW!

Imprisoning Forces

BATTLE LINE (tension, stress, pressure)

A

B

C

OBJECTIVE

Potholes in the Road

List A

I haven't been able to find a housekeeper.

I'm always exhausted.

I don't have time to investigate nursing homes.

We can't afford to hire help.

My relative can't remember anything we agree on, so talking about it is useless.

Nobody else in the family lives nearby.

There aren't any adult day care centers in our area.

My relative simply can't live alone any more; where else could he or she go?

I'm financially dependent on my relative.

I don't know how to cope with senility or depression.

I'd call to check on him, but my relative can't hear the phone.

My relative needs a special diet; Meals on Wheels doesn't have it.

I haven't been able to locate any intermediate care facilities.

My relative needs therapy three times a week and I haven't any car.

List B

I'm the logical one to provide care; everyone else in the family works.

I'm trying so hard to honor my father and my mother!

I married him, didn't I, for better or for worse.

My family just assumes I'll do it.

I really think I should do everything I possibly can to make her happy.

If my neighbor can handle caring for her relative, why can't I care for mine?

The sermon said we should be loving and sacrifice for others.

It's rude not to answer questions.

She just keeps telling us she needs family.

The hospital social worker assumes we'll take her.

My spouse thinks I ought to be doing this.

My relative thinks I have nothing else to do.

Every time I visit, my relative asks to come home with me.

My relative yells at me and has temper tantrums.

It wouldn't be respectful to order my relative around.

My relative just assumes I should do whatever he or she wants me to!

I think we should repay what our parents did for us.

My mother took care of *her* mother!

In my cultural or ethnic group, you're expected to do certain things.

List C

I promised I would take care of my relative.

I can't stand to hurt my relative's feelings.

I feel guilty that I don't really want to be so involved.

I'm afraid nobody will take care of me when I'm old.

It's just easier to let my relative have his or her own way.

I don't really want to let my sister interfere.

At last I'm in control, and my relative is going to do things *my* way!

I may not have done much with my life, but at least I can be a good caregiver.

I'm still hoping that one day, I'll get some affection back from my relative.

I'd be ashamed to admit I can't do this.

I feel guilty; after all, I moved her out of her home.

I feel so sorry for my relative!

My relative has had a really hard life; I'd like to make it up to him or her.

I'm trying to take the place of my relative's deceased spouse.

The present arrangement was a mistake, but I don't know how to say so!

I want everybody to approve of me.

I'm afraid my relative will die.

I feel guilty because I wish my relative *would* die.

I need my relative; I'd be terribly lonely without him or her.

Maybe My Partner Could...

Dispatches

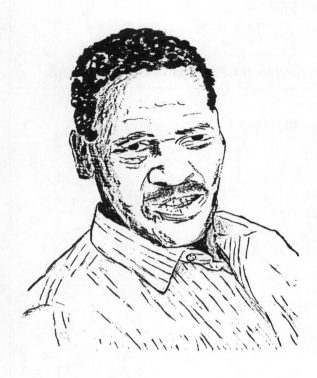

Roger:

"Not too long ago, the television program **60 Minutes** did a report on Huntington's Chorea. It showed a man in England who is spending his life caring for an afflicted wife, while his daughter grows up in a household of nothing but illness and suffering. I thought to myself, 'Huntington's Chorea is a genetic condition. It's very sad, but it's a Type 1 problem; nobody can cure his wife. Why is he hanging on and hanging on, torturing himself?'

"Then I remembered what he told the interviewer. 'Well, I married her for better or for worse.' That one quotation was keeping him from considering any other life style. He believed he had to live in the same house with her, and care for her personally, until she died."

Melissa:

"When I was in such bad shape because I couldn't get my sisters to help take care of my mother, the quotation *I* kept remembering was, "How can one mother take care of five daughters, and five daughters can't take care of one mother?"

Jane:

"With me, it was pride. If all these other people can do it, why can't I? Aren't I as good as they are?"

The Helping Process

Part A. Understand your friend's point of view and help define the problem.

1. Listen to your friend's ideas, summarize, and expand on them.

   "Tell me about it."
   "In other words, you think…"
   "What I hear you saying is…"
   "Does anything else happen that makes you think…?"

2. Accept his or her feelings.

   "I can understand that…"
   "I don't blame you for feeling…"
   "I can see that you feel really…"

3. Help to identify what's really bothering your friend.

   "The problem seems to boil down to the fact that…"
   "It looks like you're bothered by…"
   "One thing that's apparently causing trouble is…"

4. Help your friend to accept realistic limitations; point out Type 1 and Type 2 elements of the problem.

   "You really can't do anything about that part of the problem, can you?"

5. Help your friend define an ACHIEVABLE OBJECTIVE that includes what *he* or *she* is doing that contributes to the situation. Focus on Type 3 elements of the problem and on his or her goal.

   "You feel…because you…and you want…"

6. Help your friend identify the Imprisoning Forces that are holding him or her back.

   "What do you think people are expecting you to do?"
   "Do you believe….?"
   "Are you remembering a comment somebody made?"
   "Are you comparing yourself to someone?"

Part B. Develop a list of possible alternatives.

7. Ask for your friend's ideas.

   "What do you see as a good place to begin tackling this problem?"
   "What could you try to change?"

8. Begin to offer input. Ask for reactions to tentative suggestions from your own experience.

   "Do you think it might help you reach your goal if you…?"
   "Have you thought about…?"
   "What you do think would happen if…?"
   "Do you mean that if you were able to…?"
   "If you…what do you think would happen?"
   "Well, a good resource to consult for that is…"
   "You could find out more about that by…"
   "I received a lot of help from…"

9. Ask for your friend's ideas again.

   "What else could you try?"
   "Have you considered just keeping things the way they are?"
   "Are you willing to give up your goal?"

Part C. Empower your friend to act.

10. Help your friend evaluate the possible alternatives.

   "Let's look at these possibilities and see which fit in best with where you want to come out."

11. Help your friend plan and organize the steps towards his or her goal.

   "Let's see, can we list some of the things you'd need to accomplish in order to do that?"
   "Can we arrange them in some kind of order?"
   "So your first step is…"

12. Help your friend anticipate some reward when he or she follows through.

   "How will it feel to have accomplished that?"
   "How could you reward yourself?"
   "I'll be glad to talk with you again after you've done that; I want to hear how it goes."

When Your Friend Is Troubled

First reader:

Do you feel complimented when a friend asks you for help? You should. Most of us will not reveal our vulnerabilities to people we don't trust.

When a friend asks for help, he or she is saying: "I believe you care about me enough to give me your time and attention." "I believe you won't put me down just because I can't handle this problem by myself." "I believe you have the experience and skill to help me effectively."

Most of us do have experience: some knowledge of what works and what doesn't work, information about possible resources, and ideas about what could be tried. All of this is potentially valuable input. Yet if we have not learned how to be effective helpers, our wealth of suggestions may only frustrate our friend.

Second reader:

The very first, almost preliminary, thing you have to do is to get yourself "hired" as a consultant. You need to notice that your friend seems troubled and make yourself available in a non-demanding way, at the same time being willing to back off. You may say, "I notice you seem to be worried about your upcoming term paper; would you like to talk about it?" Perhaps your son replies, "Not right now." Such a response *could* be a personal rejection if you have overwhelmed him with advice in the past. But it could also just be an indication that he's working it out his own way, planning to talk it over with his teacher, or whatever. If he doesn't feel he needs you, be glad; that leaves you more energy to live your own life!

We even have to be careful about assuming that somebody *has* a problem. Maybe from his point of view, he doesn't, and he resents your implied criticism. Jane's mother-in-law had three cats who were never allowed outdoors. The odor and the kitty litter tracked through the kitchen were unbelievable, but *Nana* had no sense of smell. *Jane* had a problem (and used to bring her own meals when she visited) but Nana didn't have a problem.

Third reader:

When in doubt, *ask*. "Hey, an idea occurred to me about that project of yours; would you like to hear it?" Sadly, sometimes the people with the best ideas are the most obnoxious helpers. Don't you hate it when somebody else picks up *your* ball and runs with it?

The Same Only Different

It's a powerful feeling to realize one can help a friend solve a problem. There is, however, one little pitfall. We can get so enthusiastic we begin to think he or she has to solve it to please *us*—to prove what good helpers we are! It's even better if our friend solves his or her problem the same way we solved ours; that proves we must have been right! Be cautious. Impatience can undo the good work that has brought us this far.

Think how wonderful it feels when someone gives you the luxury of time to feel your way into a problem, time to take responsibility for it, and time to mull over possible solutions. How wonderful when my friend is there for me in my hurt *and* lets me handle it my own way!

We are all different. Our elderly relatives are different. Our family resources are different. Even if our situations appear similar on the outside, they are different on the inside. So naturally, we'll handle them differently. And that's OKAY.

In Session 7 we'll learn a technique that will help us decide which alternative is right for us.

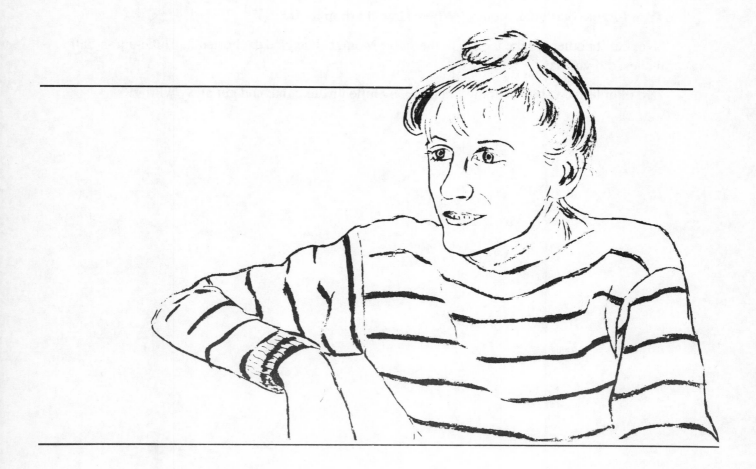

Jumping Through Hoops

When somebody else's dike develops a leak, some of us automatically rush to stick our fingers in the hole. Who depends on *you* to get them out of scrapes? Do you ever feel as if you've gotten in up to your shoulder?

This is a version of "Can You Top This." Take turns making the most outrageous "rescuing" statements you can think of. The person who gets the most laughs wins. Everyone will get a prize at the end.

Here are a few to get you started.

"Never mind, Honey. I'll call your teacher tomorrow morning."

"She invited your father to do *what*? Maybe if *I* talked to her about it..."

"Just leave this to *me; I'll* handle Mr. Petrovski!"

"I'll write a letter to Social Security, Dad. Don't worry about a thing."

"I'm going right over there and give your boss a piece of my mind!"

"You forgot your lunch money? Where should I drop it off?"

"No, don't bother to take it back to the store, Mom. I'll be glad to shorten it. Three-and-a-half inches, did you say?"

"No pimple-faced boy is going to talk to *my* little girl like that and get away with it!"

Beware These Traps

When asked for help, beware these unhelpful responses:

1. Claiming to read your friend's mind.

    "I know just how you feel."
    "I'm sure you want to…"

2. Being judgmental. Putting your friend on the defensive.

    "Boy! You really got yourself into a mess this time!"
    "Why in the world did you do that?"

3. Rejecting your friend's feelings.

    "You shouldn't get so upset."

4. Interrupting.

5. Jumping in with your own solutions.

    "My advice is to…"
    "Why don't you…"
    "What you ought to do is…"
    "You really should…"
    "For heaven's sake, don't…"

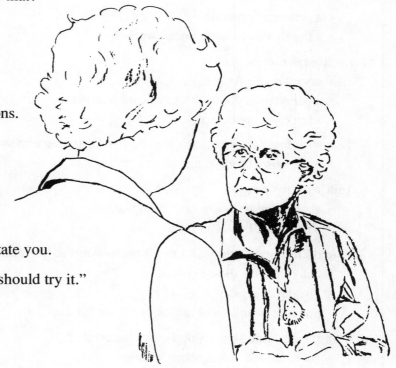

6. Assuming your friend should imitate you.

    "Well, what I did was… You should try it."

7. "Taking over" and rescuing.

    "Just let me handle this."

8. Becoming impatient.

    "You've really got to get moving!"
    "For heaven's sake, do *something!*"

9. Assuming your friend should operate from your value system.

    "Well, of course, the Bible says we ought to…"
    "The most important thing is to…"

10. Giving easy reassurance.

    "Cheer up. I'm sure everything will be okay."

Mapping Alternatives

1. Decide to leave things as they are.

2. Learn something.
- attend a seminar for families of the aged.
- read a book about coping with senility.
- take a class on Assertiveness Training.
- find out what to look for when choosing a nursing home.

3. Talk to someone with special knowledge.
- my relative's doctor.
- a geriatric specialist.
- a family counselor or social worker.

4. Locate resources.
- my relative's Area Agency on Aging.
- a geriatric diagnostic and evaluation center.
- adult day care centers.

5. Talk with family members (using Active Listening *and* statements of my own needs.)
- my spouse, brothers and sisters, children.

6. Talk with my relative.
- about what he or she needs and wants.
- about what I need and want.

7. Stop doing something that I don't really want to be doing.
- delivering meals to my relative.
- visiting every day.
- phoning at times that are inconvenient for me.

8. Stop trying to do something I can't succeed at.
- changing the nursing home routine.
- expecting my relative to remember what I tell him or her.
- getting my siblings to help more.

9. Stop permitting something that upsets me.
- allowing my relative to invite herself along on my outings.
- standing there and letting my relative "dump" on me.

10. Begin doing something that I want to do.
- arranging for household help.
- going into my bedroom and closing the door.
- starting a support group in my community.

More Alternatives

Learn something.

Talk to someone with special knowledge.

Locate resources. (See pages 4 and 5)

Stop doing something that I don't really want to be doing.

Stop trying to do something I can't succeed at.

Stop permitting something that upsets me.

Begin doing something that I want to do.

Maybe I Could...

Letters

Sabrina:

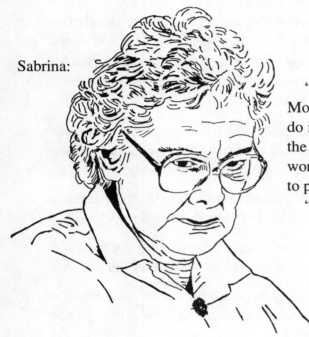

"One of the worst things is watching how exhausted my Mom is getting taking care of my Dad. She's determined to do it all herself. Oh, she'll let my sister or me come over for the afternoon, but when I suggest hiring a companion she won't hear of it. Sis and I are both working, and we'd be glad to pay for someone to come in, but that's not what they want.

"It makes it so hard to help them! All they will accept is our being there, personally, and that's the one thing we can't do. And our brother, who lives in St. Paul, can do no wrong; they think he's the perfect son. He keeps calling Sis and me telling us what to do. 'Have we gotten Dad to a ball game? Why don't we take them to Sergios for their anniversary?' He has absolutely no idea what's going on around here!

"If Gordon thinks he knows all the answers, he can quit *his* job and come get *his* hands dirty for a change!

"But being mad at Gordon doesn't help Mom. She's so determined…and so frail…it breaks my heart."

Mildred:

"When I first came to the seminar, I thought that putting Granny in a nursing home would solve all our problems. I also thought I couldn't possibly do it, because it would prove we didn't love her.

"Now that I know Bea, I realize that the nursing-home alternative only exchanges one set of problems for another set (perhaps more manageable, perhaps not).

"And I also realize that the circumstances of care have little to do with love or the lack of love. They have to do with hard physical and mental realities. Externals.

"Love is an inner gift. Nobody could love her mother more than Bea loves hers. Bea is a good daughter, and she did what had to be done. So could I. Bea would not condemn me.

"I have a friend, now, who really understands."

Judy's Story (Monologue)

Until three months ago, my mother lived with us. She required a lot of attention, but I was glad to do it, though sometimes I thought I couldn't play another game of pinochle if my life depended on it. But then I'd think, "Aren't I lucky to be able to sit here with my mother, in front of the cozy fire, and know she's well taken care of?" My husband, Herb, was really good about it. He knew I *wanted* to go on those business trips with him, even if I couldn't. And the kids cooperated, though it was hard for the three of them to get along in one bedroom. I guess we all sort of got used to arranging our lives around Mom.

At any rate, when she went to the hospital, I was surprised at how *free* we all felt. Suddenly the kids were playing their rock records and having friends sleep over. Herb and I had a dinner party! I visited the hospital every day, but compared to before, life was heavenly!

So when Mom's hip improved, we decided to try the extended care facility. We told Mom she needed the physical therapy they offer. She does. But why do I have these rotten feelings?

I go to visit, and Mom doesn't seem like my mother any more. She's in a hospital bed, with strangers all around. And she's gotten so thin and quiet. It breaks my heart to see her like that.

And she keeps asking, "Judy, when can I come home?" What can I tell her? "We don't want you at home any more, Mom?" I'm not even sure I *could* take care of her in her present condition, but I feel so guilty to think I don't want to try.

It's scary, thinking that I'll be old and dependent some day. I wonder what it will feel like, not being able to take care of myself any more, not to believe I'm going to get better. It was different when I had my foot operation; every day I felt stronger. But Mom gets weaker and weaker. I wonder what she thinks about, just lying there all day.

I've been spending every afternoon with Mom, but now Herb wants me to fly to New Orleans with him. He says *he* wants to see me sometimes, too. I don't know what to do.

I just know I'm miserable.

"Just knowing that she's miserable" doesn't give Judy a handle on her feelings. Please help sort them out. Can you identify four negative feelings she expresses?

Judy feels:

Homesickness (Interview)

What kinds of things did you and your relative enjoy that you can't do together any more?

What holidays did you celebrate together in some special way?

Did your relative have a favorite story or expression?

Recall a time your relative was the person you turned to when you needed help.

In your family's division of labor, what could you count on your relative's taking care of?

If you could give your relative back one ability, what would it be?

Do you have any regrets (or anger) about missing a quality of relationship you never had and now realize you probably never will have?

What do you want always to remember about your relative?

It's okay to mourn. Amoebas are not programmed to die. Theoretically, they could go along dividing and growing, dividing and growing, forever. A thousand years later, where would the original "grandfather amoeba" be? He'd still be alive, in a billion little bits of a billion busily-dividing, identical descendants. People are not so. Old age and death are the price we pay for our individuality. People are not interchangeable, and therefore, when time changes them, they are missed. We wouldn't want not to miss them.

Discovering What Matters to Me

My values, in order of priority, as of this date:

1st_____

2nd_____

3rd_____

4th_____

5th_____

6th_____

7th_____

8th_____

9th_____

10th_____

The Loving Thing to Do

In the long run, the most loving thing we can do for our elderly relative is to be fully ourselves. To express our own talents, give our own gifts. To pursue goals—and share the reasons they are important. To grieve losses—and share what they mean to us.

There is a hunger in the human soul that is unfed even by genuine affection. That hunger is for *intimacy.* When we reveal our true selves to others, we are making them the highest gift of all. Intimacy, by its nature, conveys trust, respect, and caring.

We have learned to Actively Listen to our relatives, grasp their hands, hug them, accept their feelings and situations. It is a loving skill. But just responding to their needs is not enough.

We are *their* creations, some of the results of their efforts. If we live restricted, frustrated lives, part of those efforts will never come to fruition.

We honor our relatives by living rich, growing, abundant lives, when we credit them with wanting rich, growing, abundant lives for us. Even if in so doing we spend less time with them. Even if in so doing we must say "no" to them. Even if in so doing we sometimes find ourselves in conflict with them.

When we are strong, when we work conflicts through, when we follow our own stars with faith and resolve—we are honoring those who produced us.

Our happiness—shared—becomes their happiness. Our success—shared—theirs. Conversely, our bitterness, unconsciously transmitted, poisons not only our souls, but theirs.

We especially feel a need to honor our parents, to care about them. Part of that honoring is *to help them be loving to us,* on whatever level they are functioning, knowing that at their best they would have given us the sun and the moon. It may mean their sharing our plans and worries. It may only mean their seeing us less often, or learning not to "dump" on us. It may mean our insisting they let go.

It is up to us to guide the relationship during these final years together. We may be the only ones who can; our relatives may no longer have the necessary range of behaviors.

Choosing a life style appropriate to our own needs is not selfish. It is fulfilling—of their lifelong care for us.

We honor our father and mother by who we are. We cannot eat for them, smile for them, breathe for them, die for them. But at the end we can help give meaning to all that has gone before.

Mary and Gram (Monologues)

The first speaker is Mary:

I'm Mary Beckman. I have an Excedrin headache. I've been having headaches a lot lately—ever since Gram came to live with us. Her arthritis is so bad, and she's so forgetful, she really can't manage alone any more. I understand that…and yet…it's awfully hard.

I remember when I used to love to have her come. One Christmas we made six kinds of cookies! But somehow, Gram has changed.

I can't even get her to take her medicine as she ought. I keep reminding her, but she's stubborn. Dr. Stevens didn't explain to her how important it is not to skip doses, and of course she won't listen to me.

It drives me crazy the way Gram has the TV on all day. Most of the time she isn't even watching it. She just seems to want the noise.

And the way she follows me around the house! If I go into my room and close the door, pretty soon she comes tap-tap-tapping, wanting to know if I'm in there. I think she really worries I'm going to vanish into thin air and leave her all alone. Sometimes I wish I could!

I mean, I have hardly any privacy at all! If my friends phone, Gram listens in on the extension. I realize she grew up with a party line, but gee whiz! I can't even have a good "gripe session."

(softer) I do realize Gram is lonely, and I do sympathize. But last night I really blew up at her. Jack and I were planning to go to the movie, and I was *so* looking forward to it. Jenny was home, working on her history paper, but guess what! By the time we got into the car, our "date" had turned into a threesome. Jack actually invited Gram to come along!

When we finally got home, I gave Gram a snack and tucked her into bed. I figured Jack and I could at least have a quiet dish of ice cream together. Would you believe Gram heard us in the kitchen and came out in her pajamas, wanting to join the party?

That did it. *"Mother!"* I screamed. *"Go back in your room and don't you dare come out again until morning!"*

Gram had such a hurt look on her face I felt just terrible. Even Jack gave me a funny look. I'll admit my ice cream didn't taste very good after that.

Fortunately, by this morning Gram seems to have forgotten all about the incident. But I haven't. I promised my father I'd always take good care of Mom…but…right now…I feel like I'm a pretty rotten daughter.

The second speaker is Mary's husband, Jack Beckman:

I'm Mary's husband, Jack. Gosh, it hurts me to see Mary so tense and miserable. I thought I was doing her a favor to let her mother come live with us.

I certainly *try* to get along with Gram. Like last night, when Gram said, "Have fun at the movie. Don't worry a bit about me…sitting here alone all evening." I knew she wanted to come along. So I invited her.

She wouldn't have been alone, actually. But Jenny was busy with her homework and not giving Gram much attention.

Anyhow, I invited her. We have a two-door car, so Gram has to sit in the front. Mary sat in the back, but—do you know—she hardly said one word all the way to the theater and back.

I wish I could fix it up so Mary could be happy again—so we all could be happy again.

The third speaker is Mary's sister, Zelda:

I'm Mary's younger sister, Zelda. I don't know how Mary stands it. Mom hangs onto her like a little kid…worse than a little kid. Of course, Mom always said Mary was the dependable one.

I'd like to be able to do more to help. My apartment doesn't have room for Mom to stay here, but I'd be glad to take her for the day now and then. Only Mom refuses to come. She doesn't like our old black-and-white TV, and she says my four-year-old twins get on her nerves. The one time she came, she was phoning Mary every five minutes to come and get her. So Mary told me not to bother inviting her anymore.

I feel guilty I'm not doing more to help.

The fourth speaker is Mary's daughter, Jenny:

I'm Jenny. I'm fourteen. Boy, is it ever a bummer to have a grandmother move in! Like…she comments on everything I do. And when my friends come over, she keeps interrupting us with a lot of silly questions. And she puts her hands all over us. Mom says Gram doesn't have many interests and we have to be polite.

But my friends haven't been coming over much lately.

I know I ought to be helping more. After all, Gram used to be one of my favorite people. I used to love to go stay overnight at *her* house. But she just won't settle down. She won't read for more than five minutes…she can't play cards…and she keeps telling me the same stories over and over.It feels like she isn't really my grandmother any more.

I'm glad they took her along last night. For once I was able to do my homework in peace. I know my grades have been slipping, but I just can't concentrate.

About the only thing Gram likes to do with me is take a walk. Mom has me go around the block with her whenever I get home from field hockey in time. I used to love going for walks, just my grandma and me. But now! You never saw anything so slow!

I wish Gram didn't have to live here.

The fifth speaker is Mary's mother, Sylvia Conwell:

I'm Mary's mother, Sylvia Conwell. I know I'm old, and I know I'm forgetful, but I think I'm entitled to a little respect.

I'm eighty-six years old, you know.

I'm no trouble to Mary, not really. I never ask her to take me any place she's not going anyhow. But I do enjoy a nice ride in the car, and there's no reason I shouldn't go along when Mary does her errands.

I'm really quite comfortable in Mary's house—except for my arthritis, that is. All my neighbors told me I was so lucky to have a family that loves me—not like that poor Mrs. Taylor, who had to go to a "home." (softer) …A "home"…

Mary agrees with me, blood is thicker than water, and there's nothing like family! Especially when all your friends are either old like you…or dead. And especially when you're eighty—what is it, five?—like I am.

{sighs) I do miss the old neighborhood, though. I even miss that big old lilac by the back door.

Of course, Mary does get a little edgy now and then. But I try to make allowances for her. Her "nerves" must be caused by those headaches she's been having.

Old Dr. Simpson would have taken care of those headaches six months ago. My arthritis, too. Those pills that young fellow gave me didn't work. I quit taking them after a couple of weeks. Just a waste of money.

I don't know what the world is coming to. You can't count on anything like you used to.

Did I tell you I'm eighty-six? It's no fun getting old….

Benefit/Cost Analysis

Consequences for:	Alternative One Leave things as they are		Alternative Two	
	Benefits	Costs	Benefits	Costs

Older person:
- safety
- nutrition
- medications
- exercise
- personal hygiene
- social contacts
- emotional welfare
- sense of control
- long-term adjustment

Me:
- time required
- health
- relationship with spouse
- relationship with children
- relationship with old person
- relationships with friends
- job/career
- travel
- sports/exercise
- education
- privacy
- hobbies
- personal freedom
- emotional welfare
- spiritual growth

My spouse:
- time required
- health
- relationship with me
- relationship with children
- relationship with old person
- relationships with friends

Consequences for:	Alternative One		Alternative Two	
	Leave things as they are			
	Benefits	**Costs**	**Benefits**	**Costs**
My spouse (continued)				
job/career				
travel				
sports/exercise				
education				
privacy				
hobbies				
personal freedom				
emotional welfare				
spiritual growth				
My children:				
time required				
relationship with parents				
relationships with siblings				
relationship with old person				
relationships with friends				
job/career				
travel				
sports/exercise				
education				
privacy				
hobbies				
personal freedom				
emotional welfare				
spiritual growth				
Family harmony:				
(relationships with my siblings, in-laws, & other relatives)				
Other Consequences:				

Judy Slices the Pie

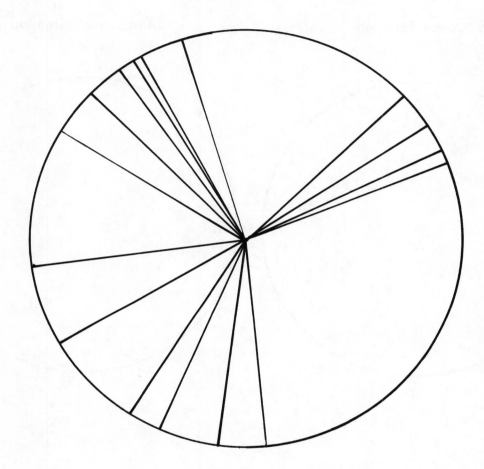

This pie represents responsibility for Judy's mother's welfare. Label each slice, choosing an appropriate-sized wedge for each person listed below. Can you think of any others? How big a slice of responsibility would you recommend Judy serve herself? Why?

doctor	Judy's children
physical therapist	Judy's brother Charles
nursing home administrator	Charles's wife Peggy
RN's at nursing home	Judy's husband Herb
dietician	Judy's Aunt Aggie (her mother's sister)
nursing assistants	Judy's mother
pastor	Judy
deacons	others?

Slicing Up My Pie

My Present Situation   **An Improved Situation**

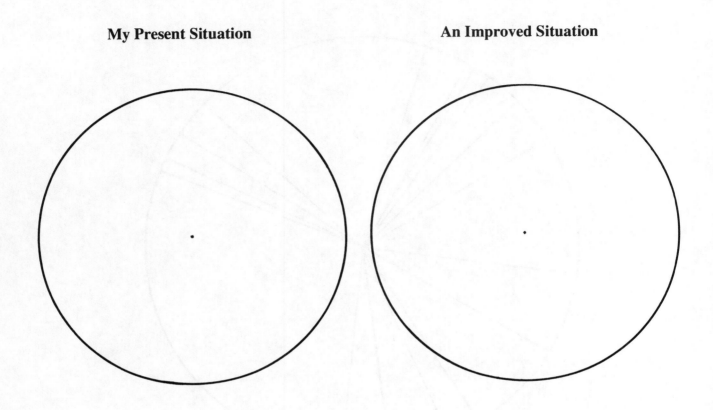

Will some of the alternatives I've been considering help me move from "here" to "there?"

How can I become more of a Care *Coordinator*?

Questions to Wrestle With

First read the page silently. Each of you is to choose one of these questions for the triad to discuss for five minutes. The three of you will probably have three different responses, and that's okay.

1. Are people who are elderly and/or ill entitled to more consideration than people who are healthy? Why or why not? If so, for how long?

2. Affirmation Nine states: "We admit that we cannot produce happiness for anyone else, including our aging loved ones." To what extent do you agree?

3. If we love others, should we try to make them happy, even if this involves taking over control of their lives?

4. Can we sometimes show love by freeing people to be themselves, even if that 'self' is depressed or cranky? How accepting should we be? How can you tell when to seek treatment and when to give up?

5. Can people give an elderly relative emotional support if they themselves are unhappy? Can a caregiver struggling with inner turmoil give peace to someone else?

6. How important is it to assure that one will have no regrets later? Do you think it is possible to guarantee this?

7. Is "Just Take One Day at a Time" an adequate response to Type 3 problems or is it better to keep trying to improve a situation? If it's better to keep trying, where can one find the energy?

8. When you become old, would you rather have a relationship of total "sweetness and light" or one that includes both light and shade, and is hence more intimate?

9. How is responsibility for an infirm spouse the same as or different from responsibility for an infirm parent?

10. Can we expect ourselves to change our feelings about a relative we never got along with just because that person is now dependent?

11. Is it helpful to try to fulfill your spouse's responsibility to his or her elderly parents—or does that keep them from developing their own relationship? Is it ever possible to "delegate" a relationship?

12. Do you think the elderly know, on some level, when we are frustrated, angry or discouraged? Is it possible to hide our feelings from people who know us so well?

The Compass Points Home

When we are in doubt about a decision, we may want to ask ourselves, "Which course of action will increase the amount of love in the world?" If we try caring for an elderly relative in a certain way—even a way our culture approves—and find ourselves feeling burdened and resentful, maybe we'd better look again. That burdensome feeling is not a sign we're bad. It's a compass, telling us we're off course.

As human beings, we operate on trial and error. A past decision doesn't have to commit us for the rest of our lives. We can say, "I thought I could…but I didn't know…; my decision led to something different from what I expected…."

There aren't any perfect solutions. Furthermore, love is different from achievement. We may even be surprised to discover that modifying stressful circumstances permits love to *grow*.

Our relationship with our elderly relatives is in flux. It will continue to be in flux. Even if *they* don't change, *we* change. We're allowed to get tired. Allowed to change our minds. Allowed to try something new. Allowed to ask for help. Going on with our lives is okay.

Suddenly Rachel Took Charge

Margaret:

"When I talked to my friend Rachel I found she was in a much worse situation than I was! Her mother was an absolute tyrant—always had been. Rachel would come home from work to hear, "The trouble with you is, you're lazy." Rachel's house was overflowing with Mother's furniture. Mother's demands drove everybody crazy.

"One day, as we were crying on each other's shoulders, I told my friend, "Rachel, I just know something is going to happen to change your life. I don't know what it is, but watch for it."

"Some months later, Rachel called and reminded me of that conversation. Something *had* happened. Rachel's husband had had a heart attack. *Of course* Rachel couldn't take care of both of them. In four days Mother was back upstate!

"It took a calamity to give Rachel permission to meet her own needs.

"I wonder if Rachel's mother is benefitting from the opportunity to learn other ways of relating to people. I hope so.

"Why couldn't Rachel take action before? I suspect she'd been taught that if we love someone, we ought to make her happy—that is—DO WHAT SHE WANTS. Quite an Imprisoning Force to overcome, isn't it?"

Do I Want to Change?

Read the following common situations. Put a check (√) by responses you have given in the past. Put a plus (+) by responses you want to use in the future. (Perhaps some of them will be the same.)

1. When there's a choice between spending an afternoon doing what I *want* to do and what I think I *should* do:
   _____ I generally believe in spinach first and hope I'll get ice cream later.
   _____ I usually choose whatever offers more immediate pleasure.
   _____ I try to figure out a way to do both.
   _____ I get frustrated and confused and end up doing neither.
   _____ Whichever I choose, I don't enjoy it.
   _____ Other:

2. When there's a difference between what *I* want to do and what someone else wants to do:
   _____ I'm easily talked into going along, and usually end up enjoying it.
   _____ I go along to keep the peace, but resent it.
   _____ I try to negotiate.
   _____ Other:

3. When there's a hard decision to be made:
   _____ I postpone it.
   _____ I make it quickly to get it over with.
   _____ I wait for someone else to make it.
   _____ I plan when and how I'm going to decide and begin gathering facts.
   _____ Other:

4. When I'm having difficulty with something:
   _____ I tell my friends about it.
   _____ I don't want my friends to know.
   _____ I ask for help.
   _____ I resist asking for help.
   _____ I hope I can muddle through.
   _____ I give up.
   _____ I keep struggling and striving to resolve the problem.
   _____ Other:

5. When deciding how to respond to a request for a favor, my principal concern is:
   _____ avoiding disapproval.
   _____ figuring out how I really feel about it.
   _____ Other:

The Fork in the Trail

We are nearer to defining what *we* want, but of course our elderly relatives have wants and needs, too. What if our needs conflict? Am I supposed to ignore the needs of others and just take care of my own? Or vice versa? What happens if I don't take responsibility for improving my own life and remain a victim? Well, there are some advantages to that. I avoid risks. I stay weak. I don't have to keep trying. I have somebody or some situation to blame. I avoid having to change. I avoid confrontation. I continue getting approval. I avoid pain, *except the pain I carry with me all the time*.

What happens if I accept responsibility for seeing that both my elderly relative's needs and my own needs are met? THEN I CAN FULFILL THAT RESPONSIBILITY IN WHATEVER WAYS SEEM BEST TO ME.

Stepping Stones

Tell your partner about the alternative you have chosen to work on. Unless you have decided to leave things as they are, you'll need to do many things to implement it. Your first task is to make a list of all necessary steps. Your partner will help you think of them. Your second task is to number the steps in "tackling order." Sometimes it helps to undertake the easiest first!

Chosen Alternative:

My Stepping Stones:

Caregiving Changes Us

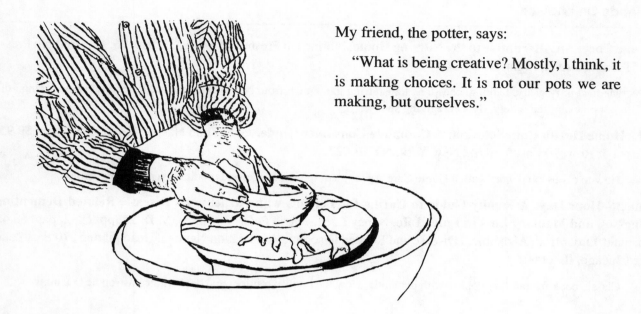

My friend, the potter, says:

"What is being creative? Mostly, I think, it is making choices. It is not our pots we are making, but ourselves."

"There is an energy within each of us that has to be used, and we learn about ourselves as well as about the energies of others when we tap into that energy in new ways. The first thing a potter does when working on the wheel is to center the clay...bring it in tight and push in rhythm until a bumpy lump is brought into a smoothly-spinning sphere...right in the center of the wheel in perfect balance. Lots of people use this image to describe getting one's life in order...getting on center...pulling yourself together...getting a grasp on things. But that is just the first step. For after I center the clay, if I leave it that way, all together in perfect harmony, what happens? Nothing. It just sits there spinning.

"To make a pot I have to make a hole and then gently but firmly pull it off center...and up. That is how a pot grows, and that is how we grow. By stepping off the safe ground where the ball is predictably going around and around and taking a chance that maybe we'll make a pot.

"For a potter, the big risk comes when she puts the finished pot—that she worked so hard on—into the kiln. Without firing, it will stay intact, but worthless.

"If one fires in a simple, home-made sawdust kiln, the results are unpredictable. Sometimes the mottled grays and blacks are not to our taste, and we have to start over. But sometimes the finished pot has striking beauty, an unexpected pattern and coloration produced by its ordeal in the heat.

"Potters call it 'The Gift of the Fire.'"

Good Reading for Caregivers

"Hands On" Advice

Home Care: An Alternative to the Nursing Home. Florine Du Fresne. 127pp. 1983. pap. $6.95.. Brethren Press, 1451 Dundee Ave., Elgin, IL 60120.

Medical nitty-gritty: bathing, bedsores, transferring the patient from bed to chair and back, record keeping, range-of-motion exercises, safety. By a caregiving spouse.

The Home Health Care Solution: A Complete Consumer Guide. Janet Zhun Nassif. 416pp. 1985. pap. $9.95. Harper & Row, 10 East 53rd St., New York, NY 10022.

How to choose and work with a Home Care Agency, equip your home, and monitor agency supervision.

The 36–Hour Day: A Family Guide to Caring for Persons with Alzheimer's Disease, Related Dementing Illnesses, and Memory Loss in Later Life. Nancy L. Mace and Peter V. Rabins, M.D. 253pp. 1982. pap. $8.45 postpaid. Order from Alzheimers Disease and Related Disorders Association National Headquarters, 70 East Lake St., Chicago, IL 60601.

Classic book for families coping with dementia. How to simplify routines and deal with catastrophic reactions.

Planning

Care–Giving: Helping an Aging Loved One. Jo Horne. 318pp. 1985. pap. $13.95. AARP Books, Scott, Foresman and Co., 400 S. Edward St., Mt. Prospect, IL 60056.

Begins with the basic question: Should you become a caregiver? Decision-making. Meeting the needs of the care recipient and the caregiver. Dealing with difficult feelings.

Legal/Financial Planning Guide for Families. Tim Nay. 87pp. 1987. pap. $15 postpd. Good Samaritan Hospital & Medical Center, 1040 NW 22nd St., Portland, OR 97210.

Step-by-step planning when long-term care is anticipated. Protecting the financial security of the unimpaired. Valuable!

Supportive Living Arrangements for Older Citizens: A Guide. Anneta S. Kraus, R.N. 45pp. 1984. pap. $4.00 + $1.00 postage. Geriatric Planning Services, Mainline Federal Bldg., #201, Front and Orange Sts., Media, PA 19063.

Housing and care options described by an expert . How a family conference can help members cooperate in care.

Relationships

How to Tape Instant Oral Biographies, 3rd, rev. ed. William Zimmerman. 112pp. 1982 pap. $4.95 + $1.00 shipping. Guarionex Press Ltd., 201 West 77th St., New York, NY 10024.

Directions for interviewing older relatives. Questions to ask. Jogging memories. Guaranteed to deepen relationships.

Mainstay: A Companion Guide for the Spouses of the Chronically Ill. Maggie Strong. 352pp. 1988. $17.95 Little, Brown and Company, 34 Beacon St., Boston, MA 02106.

> The effect changed dependencies can have on an entire family. How to survive the long haul. While primarily addressed to the middle-aged or younger, the book speaks to well spouses of any age.

Talking With Your Aging Parents. Mark A. Edinberg. 220pp. 1987. hardback $16.95. Shambhala Publications, Inc., 314 Dartmouth Street, Boston, MA 02116.

> How to discuss important issues—housing, legal and financial planning, health, confusion, nursing homes, family matters, your own life style—with older parents. Dealing with guilt, avoidance, denial, manipulation, and sabotage.

For Those From Dysfunctional Families Who Are Now Caring for a Parent

Adult Children of Alcoholics. Janet Woititz. 106pp. 1983. pap. $6.95. Health Communications, Inc., 1721 Blount Rd., Suite 1, Pompano Beach, FL 33069.

> Why you may be too hard on yourself, feel compelled to control others, or take impulsive action without considering long-range consequences. Not written for caregivers, but useful if you grew up in any kind of dysfunctional family.

About Nursing Home Placement

Caring Relationships: Guide for Families of Nursing Home Residents. Hope Cassidy and Linda Flaherty. 24pp. 1982. pap. $2.50 + $.50 postage. Augsburg Publishing House, 426 S. Fifth St., Minneapolis, MN 55415.

> Accepting change. Adjusting to a new lifestyle. Grief. Offering choices. Coping with misdirected anger. Supporting the withdrawn. Living with hearing and vision impairments or speech barriers. Empathetic listening. Beautiful, cogent booklet.

Choosing a Nursing Home: A Guidebook for Families. Marty Richards, Nancy Hooyman et al. 110pp. 1985. pap. $8.95. University of Washington Press, P.O. Box C-50096, Seattle, WA 98145-5096.

> How to tell when it's time to seek a nursing home. The feasibility of a person's living alone or coming into one's own home. Adjustment of all family members to a placement decision.

What Do I Do? How to Care for, Comfort, and Commune with Your Nursing Home Elder. Katherine L. Karr. 130pp. Rev. ed. 1985. $14.95 Haworth Press, Inc., 28 East 22 Street, New York, NY 10010-6194.

> Physical, Emotional, Mental, and Spiritual Care. Each section includes detailed checklists with practical suggestions for monitoring and supplementing care. Sensitive and realistic. This is the book I want my children to read when I'm in a nursing home.

When Love Gets Tough: The Nursing Home Decision. Rev. ed. Doug Manning. 91pp. 1983. pap. $5.00, postpaid. In-Sight Books, Inc., P.O. Box 2058, Hereford, TX 79045.

> "I dream of great loads of guilt being laid aside…of residents beginning to understand their own feelings and the feelings of others…of families and nursing homes becoming care teams." The most complete description we have seen of the adjustment process new residents go through and how to assist them.

Manna for the Wilderness

Session 1: Adjusting to Aging

Scripture: *"Bear one another's burdens..."* Galatians 6:2

"For everything there is a season and a time for every matter under heaven: a time to be born, and a time to die...." Ecclesiastes 3:1-2

Thought: We are different from each other in many ways and our elderly relatives have different needs, but we are united in the determination to provide for their welfare. What a relief it is to share feelings! What hope it gives to discover that others understand what we are going through and believe we can learn to cope!

Prayer: Lord, thank you for bringing this group together. Send your Holy Spirit to participate with us. Be with each family represented here in the weeks ahead. Amen.

Session 2: Learning to Listen

Scripture: *"Rejoice with those who rejoice; weep with those who weep."* Romans 12:15

"Then children were brought to him that he might lay his hands on them and pray... And he laid his hands on them...." Matthew 19:13a,15

"And this is the confidence which we have in him, that if we ask anything according to his will he hears us." I John 5:14

Thought: The thought that *God* Actively Listens to us—that he wants us to share our *feelings* with him—may be a new idea. But Jesus called us friends, and friends listen without judging. They touch and bless.

Prayer: Lord, it is so wonderful that you have given us speech with which to share and ears with which to listen. I confess there are some people I don't really want to hear. Let me know when you want me to pay attention. Give us all a chance to use our new skill and help us do it correctly. Amen.

Session 3: Which Problems Can I Solve?

Scripture: *"...my soul is bereft of peace, I have forgotten what happiness is;"*
Lamentations 3:17

"I will give free utterance to my complaint; I will speak in the bitterness of my soul. I will say to God...Does it seem good to thee to oppress?" Job 10:1b,c,2a,3a

"Be strong, and let your heart take courage, all you who wait for the Lord!"
Psalm 31:24

Thought: It's okay to complain loudly to God, to question God, to be angry with God. Honest communication is the only foundation for a relationship, and God wants a relationship with us! Sometimes it seems as if nothing is happening, but it is. God always hears and wants the best for everyone in any situation. Maybe a changed perspective is the prerequisite for the resolution of problems.

Prayer: Lord, we're getting down to the nitty-gritty. I don't know what's best for the families represented in this group. But *you* do. I lift all of our elderly relatives and ourselves up to your love. Please, when you give any instructions, make them so clear that we can follow them with complete confidence. Amen.

Session 4: Why Do I Feel Stuck?

Scripture: *"When Jesus saw his mother, and the disciple whom he loved standing near, he said to his mother, 'Woman, behold your son!' Then he said to the disciple, 'Behold, your mother!' And from that hour the disciple took her to his own home." John 19:26-27*

"For this is the love of God, that we keep his commandments. And his commandments are not burdensome." I John 5:3

Thought: Jesus gave *his* mother into the care of others. He didn't say, "Sorry, Father, I can't fulfill your plan for my life; I have to take care of my mother." On the contrary, he said, "He who loves father or mother more than me is not worthy of me." (Matthew 10:37) It's pretty clear that we are not to make filial love into an idol. We are to love God and hold ourselves ready to receive marching orders.

Prayer: Lord, you've promised that wherever your spirit is, there is freedom. I claim freedom from cultural assumptions and expectations for the people in this group. Blow through our minds this week. Blow away any cobwebs that are keeping us from hearing your voice and yours alone. Amen.

Session 5: How to Help a Friend

Scripture: *"A friend loves at all times...."* Proverbs 17:17

"...Julius treated Paul kindly, and gave him leave to go to his friends and be cared for." Acts 27:3

"...Cast the net on the right side of the boat...." John 21:6

Thought: What a blessing to have friends who care for us! Jesus also has called us friends and cares for us. Like any other good friend, he doesn't claim to read our minds, is not judgmental, does not reject our feelings or interrupt, and is not impatient. And he doesn't jump in and rescue us. Sometimes we wish he would! But Jesus doesn't want weak, dependent, incapable friends. He wants us to grow into mature adults who are capable of helping bring in the Kingdom. He does make suggestions sometimes, when we ask for them. They may seem to require us to go out on a limb; he always goes with us.

Prayer: Lord, you're opening up possibilities, right here in this room. It's exciting to watch. Make us wise as serpents and gentle as doves. Stay very close this week. Provide the new ideas *you* have in mind and the courage to try them. Amen.

Session 6: Heartache and Healing

Scripture: *"You shall have no other gods before me."* Exodus 20:3

"The kingdom of heaven is like a treasure hidden in a field, which a man found and covered up; then in his joy he goes and sells all that he has and buys that field." Matthew 13:44

Thought: It's okay to put all your eggs in one basket—so long as that basket represents the Kingdom of Heaven. But, like other precious things, God's plan for our life may be hidden. When we persist in a lifestyle chosen because it was the "obvious thing to do," we may miss the treasure. It's worth a lot of digging to discover God's will.

Prayer: Oh, Lord, it's so hard to believe that you want *me* to be happy. I always thought you wanted to *use* me to make *other people* happy. I can hardly believe you want me to fulfill all those talents and longings in my own heart—though I guess you must have put them there. Help all of us here believe that you really do love us, too. Amen.

Session 7: Trusting My Decisions

Scripture: *"For which of you, desiring to build a tower, does not first sit down and count the cost, whether he has enough to complete it?" Luke 14:28*

"Honor your father and your mother, that your days may be long in the land which the Lord your God gives you." Exodus 20:12

"So whatever you wish that men would do to you, do so to them; for this is the law and the prophets." Matthew 7:12

"Therefore, my beloved...work out your own salvation with fear and trembling; for God is at work in you, both to will and to work for his good pleasure. Do all things without grumbling or questioning...." Philippians 2:12–14

Thought: What land has God given to each of us? What hopes, interests, education, talents, career, abilities, spouse, children...? Finding a way to assure care for our relatives *and at the same time* to claim the blessings God has in mind for ourselves is an awesome responsibility. This is no time for snap judgments. We are required to grapple with circumstances, balancing and harmonizing interests so that we will be *able* to provide care without grumbling or questioning.

"Is not this the fast that I choose...to undo the thongs of the yoke, to let the oppressed go free...to share your bread with the hungry, and bring the homeless poor into your house; when you see the naked, to cover him, and not to hide yourself from your own flesh? Then shall your light break forth like the dawn, and your healing shall spring up speedily; your righteousness shall go before you....Then you shall call, and the Lord will answer; you shall cry, and he will say, Here I am....And the Lord will guide you continually, and satisfy your desire with good things, and make your bones strong; and you shall be like a watered garden, like a spring of water, whose waters fail not. Isaiah 58:6-11 (portions)

The one thing we are not allowed to do is turn our backs upon our elderly relatives. We are required to act responsibly. When we do, God will stay involved. Guidance comes in many ways: through scripture, through reading or conversation, through circumstance and coincidence,. Sometimes it comes as an inner calm that assures us—even in the midst of problems—that we are on the right track. If we ask for guidance, intending to obey, it always comes. God will not leave us comfortless.

Prayer: Lord, you are so great, and I know so little of your power. Teach me to listen for your guidance and recognize it. Then give me courage to obey. Help us all trust you more. Amen.

Session 8: Fulfilling My Responsibility

Scripture: *"He leads me in paths of righteousness." Psalm 23:3*

"I will be the God of all the families...and they shall be my people. The people who survived...[have] found grace. I have loved you with an everlasting love; therefore I have continued my faithfulness to you. Again I will build you, and you shall be built....Give praise and say, 'The Lord has saved his people.' Jeremiah 31:1–7 (Portions)

He is like a tree planted by streams of water, that yields its fruit in its season, and its leaf does not wither. In all that he does, he prospers." Psalm 1:3

"Do not be conformed to this world but be transformed by the renewal of your mind, that you may prove what is the will of God.... Romans 12:2

Thought: Those who learn to trust God can give up the need for approval and rely on his mercy instead. We won't always be right, but we'll always be loved.

Prayer: Lord, thank you for the fellowship of this group and for participating with us. Bless us all as we continue our separate pilgrimages. Bless our families. Stay near. Amen.

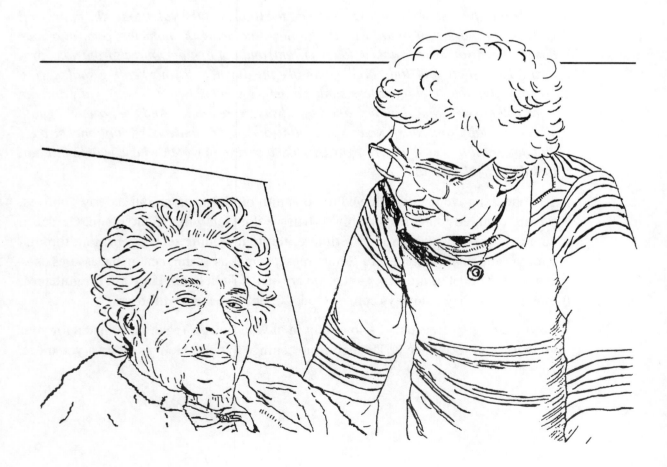

ORDER BLANK

To: SUPPORT SOURCE   Telephone (215) 544-3605
420 Rutgers Avenue, Suite 2
Swarthmore, PA 19081

Please send the following books. We understand that we may return any book for a full refund at any time.

[   ] **Help for Families of the Aging: Leader's Manual** $39.95 $ _____

2-5 copies, $31.95 ea.

(Placing your order with a co-leader saves money for both of you.)

[   ] **Help for Families of the Aging: Workbook** $11.95 $ _____

2-5 copies, $9.50 ea.; 6-10, $8.35 ea.; 11-25, $7.17 ea.

SUBTOTAL FOR BOOKS $ _____

Pennsylvanians: Please add 6% sales tax $ _____
or give us your tax-exempt number. _____

Shipping: Please add $2.00 for the first book and 50c for each additional book $ _____

GRAND TOTAL—CHECK ENCLOSED, payable to Support Source $ _____

All orders must include payment or authorized agency purchase order.

Organization _____

Name _____

Address _____

_____
                                        ZIP